NeuroCranial Restructuring: Unleash Your Structural Power

By Dean Howell, N.D.

HOWELL CANYON PRESS
P.O. BOX 448
TONASKET, WASHINGTON 98855

2000
ISBN 1-931210-02-0

ACKNOWLEDGEMENTS

There are many people whom I would like to thank for their assistance with the making of this book--

I would like to thank my wife Trisha for her writing, editing and her service as a sounding board for my sometimes too-wild ideas.

Thanks go to all the members of the NeuroCranial Restructuring Doctors' Association for their continuing efforts to apply NCR in their practices to serve mankind.

And for insisting that I print (and helping to pay for) this third edition of the book thanks to Lewis Arrandt, DC, my stalwart helper in many NCR endeavors; Douglas Hays, DC, my earliest student still current with this technique, James Sensenig, ND and Boyer Cole, NMD, the original naturopathic physicians to use this therapy, Charles Musich, DC, and Adam Del Torto, DC, the enthusiastic Californians and my golf buddy Dean Odmark, DC (may the eyes of Texas be upon you!).

Thanks to my daughter Selena, whose faith and trust in me creates her confidence in dealing with my patients with tact, sensitivity and honesty.

Thanks to my therapists/assistants Hillary Lampers, Trisha Howell and Nathan DeTracy, because they have learned to tolerate my methodology changing with every treatment sequence.

To my patients, thank you for persevering as I occasionally fumble while trying to improve this unusual therapy.

Dean Howell, ND
September 2000

TABLE OF CONTENTS

Introduction
—by Dean Howell, ND
Page 9

Getting NeuroCranial Restructuring Is Like Repairing the Structure of a Building
—by Trisha Howell
Page 11

Answers to Frequently Asked NCR Questions

By Dean Howell, ND
Page 14

I. Philosophy of NCR **Page 14**

What is NCR?
How does NCR represent a new paradigm shift in healing?
Why aren't good diet, exercise and rest enough to correct all my health problems and to optimize my structure?
Why does NCR help so many diverse conditions?
How do you know NCR works?

II. General Information **Page 16**

Can everyone benefit from NCR?
How many treatments do I need? Why do some people need more treatments than others do?
Do a lot of people return for further treatment?
How long does each treatment take?
Why do you schedule treatments four days in a row? Is there a limit to how many treatments I should get in a row? How long should I wait between sequences?
Why do you take pictures before and after each series?
How long can I keep getting benefits from each treatment series and from NCR in general?
How long after having a fracture to my nose can I begin treatment? What are the precautions in treating me?

What are the youngest and the oldest ages of people you can treat with NCR?
Will I feel okay to go out to eat after a treatment? What about eating before my treatment?
Do other doctors practice NCR?
Who is eligible to be trained as a NCR therapist? How long does the initial training take and what does it cost?
What's involved in my being a patient for a student doctor during one of the NCR training courses? How much does it cost to be seen by a student doctor?

III. Anatomy, Structure and NCR Page 22

Why does my spine and whole nervous system shift from moving my head?
What causes my cranial bones to become unbalanced in the first place?
How does moving my sphenoid move all the other cranial bones?
How can my skull, which is made of bone, expand and contract?
How do my neurotransmitter levels change from receiving treatment?
Can NCR prevent or reverse age-related stooping?

IV. NCR Technique Page 27

How do you diagnose how many balloons to use and where?
What happens when the balloons are inflated?
What does depth of balloons mean?
Why is there a special massage before the balloons?
Why do you place my body in a special position during treatment?
Is there anything I can do to accelerate my progress with NCR?
Is there anything that impedes my progress with NCR? What should I avoid?

V. NCR vs. Other Therapies Page 31

What makes NCR different from all other therapies?
How is NCR different from craniosacral therapy?

Can I have NCR in place of some dental work? How long after treatment should I wait to have dental work done? What is the proper protocol for dental work with NCR?
Why does my spine keep going back into a painful position after chiropractic adjustments and how is NCR different?
Is NCR more effective cosmetically than plastic surgery?

VI. Effects and Results of NCR Page 34

Does treatment hurt?
Can I function normally right after a treatment?
Might I vomit or have a toxic release after treatment?
What should I do if I easily bleed, bruise or am on blood thinners?
What if I have a tendency to blackout?
How does NCR affect pregnant and delivering women? Are there any precautions?
How does NCR affect athletic performance?
How long does my head keep shifting after treatment?
What happens if I keep getting treatments after my symptoms disappear? What does NCR do besides relieving conditions and these symptoms? Can I grow as a person from NCR? How?
Does NCR have any bad side effects?
What are some good NCR side effects?
Why do I feel clearer, calmer and happier after receiving NCR treatment?
Why does my face change shape with treatment? Why does it tend to become more oval and symmetrical?
How do vitamins and minerals flow after treatment? Might I need to change my supplement dosages? Why?
What do I do if I get a strange reaction between sequences?
Why does my nose sometimes run or bleed after getting treatment?
Why do my teeth sometimes ache after treatment?
Why do my feet and arches look different after treatment?

VII. NCR Answers to Conditions Page 41

What is the protocol for comatose patients?
Why does NCR treatment--which is structural--seem to help some of my biochemical problems such as poor digestion and post-nasal drip?

How and why does NCR help the following conditions? Page 41
Alzheimer's?
Anxiety and nervousness?
Arthritis, bursitis and rheumatism?
Attention Deficit Disorder, dyslexia, hyperactivity and other learning disabilities?
Autism?
Brain surgery?
Cerebral palsy?
Bipolar disorder (Manic-depression)? Depression? Obsessive-compulsive disorder?
Psychosis? Schizophrenia?
Concussion and other head injuries?
Down's Syndrome?
Dystonia?
Ear infection (acute and chronic otitis media) and deafness?
Forty-seven chromosome individuals?
Glaucoma? Double vision? Other vision problems? Headaches, head pressure and migraines?
Heart conditions?
Insomnia?
Low energy (fibromyalgia, chronic fatigue)?
Lymphatic circulation and its malfunctioning, such as lymphoma, lymphatic toxins and lymphoid?
TMD or TMJ (Mouth, head and jaw pains)?
Multiple sclerosis and amyotrophic lateral sclerosis (Lou Gehrig's disease)?
Muscular dystrophy?
Muscle spasms?
Neck and shoulder pain?
Organ functioning?
Orthodontic stress and bruxism (grinding)?
Osteoporosis?
Para- and quadriplegics?
Parkinson's disease and tremors?
Phobias?
Polio?
Poor concentration and focus?
Relationship difficulties?

Sciatica, kyphosis (hunchback), lordosis (swayback), scoliosis (a spiral spine), military spine (from whiplash) and other back problems?
Seizures?
Sinusitis? Sleep apnea? Snoring?
Breathing and sinus disorders?
Strokes? Thrombosis (excessive blood clotting)?
Left hemisphere paresis?
Tinnitus?
Tuberculosis?
Vertigo and other balance problems?

An Extract of a Report to An Attorney

by Dean Howell, ND

Page 71

NCR Testimonials

Page 74

Here's My Story: Sleep Apnea Cured **Page 74**
—Phillip Rogers
Let's Get Our Heads On Straight **Page 77**
—Marge Hartwig
My Scoliosis Is Going Away **Page 79**
—Ginny Stafford
With NCR I Can Realize My Full Potential
Page 81
—Trisha Howell, BA, MA, MA, MA
My Tensions Came From My Scoliosis
Page 83
—Anna Bond

My Ankylosing Spondylitis Got Better With NCR
Page 84
—Jamie Cuddihy
NCR Helped My Son's Hyperactivity and Learning Disabilities **Page 89**
—Susan Casey

My Down's Syndrome Daughter Gets Better and Better
Page 92
—Anna Bond

My Bizarre, But Phenomenal Healing Experience **Page 94**
—Ginger Chalford, Ph.D.
NCR for Newborns **Page 104**
—Trisha Howell

NEUROCRANIAL RESTRUCTURING!?

WHAT'S THAT?

Here is a collection of writings about NeuroCranial Restructuring (NCR), the newest and most powerful concept of physical medicine in the world today. Although rough around the edges, this small book should help you gain some understanding of this exciting foray into new ideas in physical medicine therapies.

As you read through this book, please be aware of the shortcomings of physical medicine treatments as they are practiced today. Chronic conditions are the bread and butter of the physical medicine industry. Patients believe that they cannot get better, so they accept palliative care, insuring that they will be permanent customer/patients. My frustration with ineffective therapy was the initial push to create *NeuroCranial Restructuring*.

NCR is a cumulative manipulation process involving controlled release of the body's connective tissue tension to unwind the structure and return it towards its original design. NCR utilizes careful analysis of the body's proprioception (patterns of balance) to determine the precise areas of the skull needing to be unlocked. The skull is actually moved by the action of small, inflatable endonasal balloons that are inserted through the nostril and inflated briefly into the throat.

With the addition of careful body positioning to increase the tension in the meninges and other connective tissues, the entire skeletal structure can be permanently changed with this kind of skull manipulation. This unlocking of the connective tissues' residual tensions combined with precise movements of the cranial bones allow the structural systems of the body to move incrementally and cumulatively towards the body's original design.

This has become my life's work. I hope that you become as excited by this information as I am.

All of the mistakes contained in this book are mine. There are many people who have helped, especially those people who have contributed articles and allowed their less-than-flattering photos to be published. Special thanks go to my patients for enduring my tardiness starting my workday because of my time writing this book, and my family, especially my wife Trisha, for enduring my late nights.

Dean Howell, ND
September 6, 1998

Getting NeuroCranial Restructuring Is Like Repairing The Structure of a Building

by Trisha Howell

Imagine a building made of the finest materials and impeccably maintained. Nevertheless, it constantly develops cracks and leaks. Even the most meticulously installed features crumble. All because the overall structure—the skeleton of the building—is faulty.

In the human body we often forget the importance of structure. We exercise, diet, cleanse, get good nutrition and rest. But for many of us this isn't enough because the mechanics of our bodies are not working at their peak.

Starting with the birthing process, our heads are squeezed and compressed into less than their optimal shapes. Each time we receive a physical or emotional blow to the skull, the sutures—the cranial bone joints—tighten and put pressure on the brain, diminishing optimal learning and well-being. The skull distorts, which in turn distorts the spine, pelvis, legs and feet, producing anything from minor dysfunction to great pain.

The body's structural priority is stability, keeping the person upright and balanced. If the head is even slightly distorted, then it doesn't balance easily, and the spine compensates with a counterbalancing distortion to create a makeshift stability.

This is why so many chiropractic adjustments to the spine don't hold—the spine's distortion, though painful, is more functional and stabilizing to the head than the adjusted position. So the body returns to its compensatory pattern.

Likewise, in many cases massage is unable to provide long-term relief to achy muscles because the muscles' tension is more functional. When the structure is unbalanced and unable to properly support itself, stability is gained by muscle tension. The muscles are like cables holding up a tree—you don't want to loosen them or the tree will fall over. The tree must first be restored to a healthy structure.

This is much easier to do for the human body than for a tree. It's possible to unlock the sutures in the skull so that the brain has room to operate efficiently and the entire nervous system is optimized. The only therapy currently available that makes positive and permanent structural change from the head down is NeuroCranial Restructuring (NCR).

NCR moves the head and entire body more and more towards its original design. The face becomes more symmetrical, the head rounder, the posture and movement more graceful and easy. This increased stability is effortless for the patient—one naturally stands straighter and more balanced when the structure is optimized.

NCR works by moving the sphenoid bone, the foundation for all the other bones in the head. When the sphenoid is off, so is everything else. When the sphenoid is properly balanced, everything else can be optimized too.

With NCR, the cranial bones relax, returning to their originally design and shape, allowing the brain to fully expand. With the head properly shaped and positioned, the spine naturally returns to its optimal shape and function. Muscular tension disappears because it is no longer required for stability. Flexibility and ease of movement return. Increased energy and a profound sense of well being arise.

Dr. Dean Howell, the founder of NCR therapy, and the doctors he's trained, perform an external examination to test the sphenoid's stability. Depending on where and how much it is unstable, they design a pattern of treatment tailored to the individual. Small balloons of varying thickness are inserted into one to four of the six nasal passages to the throat, permitting a momentary direct contact with the sphenoid bone. The patient's body positions during treatment are also determined with this testing. One or two persons will be instructed by the doctor in precise patterns of holding the body to immobilize the body to maximize the change that the body is able to make. Then the balloon is inflated from two to five seconds to precisely move the sphenoid and thus all the other cranial bones, creating a new and superior stability. For maximal results, the patient receives one treatment a day over four consecutive days.

Dr. Howell has personally administered over 60,000 treatments. They have been safe and highly effective in reducing or eliminating symptoms as diverse as breathing and sinus dysfunction, muscular pain and spasm, scoliosis, ear disorders, vision problems, seizures, whiplash, dyslexia, insomnia, snoring, sleep apnea, dystonia, Parkinson's tremors and TMJ.

NCR also has profound mental and emotional effects, including relief from anxiety, depression, phobias, hyperactivity, nervousness and even lessening of the symptoms of Down's Syndrome and Alzheimer's. Patients report feeling more relaxed, happy and self-confident. Creativity is enhanced. Relationships improve. Learning becomes easier. Concentration, focus, mental and emotional clarity all increase.

The variety and intensity of positive physical, mental and emotional effects from optimizing the body's structure through NCR are astounding. This demonstrates that the body's structural integrity is far more important than we normally realize. Together with proper diet, exercise and rest, good structure is the key to the body, mind and emotions operating at their full potential.

NCR is the only therapy that moves the sphenoid bone—and with it, the entire structure—precisely and effectively. If we want to be the best we can be both individually and societally, receiving NCR is the place to start.

I. Philosophy of NCR

What is NCR?

NeuroCranial Restructuring is a manipulation process used to unwind the body into its original and optimal design. It utilizes careful analysis of the body's proprioception (patterns of balance) to determine the precise areas of the skull needing to be unlocked. This unlocking allows the connective tissues (including the meningeal system) to release their residual tensions and move the bony structures incrementally back towards the body's original design.

How does NCR represent a new paradigm shift in healing?

In traditional natural medicine, the emphases in healing are placed on detoxification of metals, chemicals and toxins, hygienic living and removal of infective organisms. Except for recovery from accidents and injuries, the physical medicine techniques like massage, physiotherapy and manipulation are used for pain relief. To accomplish this, a patient comes in on a regular schedule. There can be some long-term improvements, but they are generally local changes like a lessening of the intensity of headaches or neck pain.

With NCR, long-term changes are the normal response, and the eventual result is an optimization of nervous system functions. What I have found is that many conditions thought to be biochemical, developmental or infective in nature have a previously unknown, correctable structural component. This means that conditions like Alzheimer's, Parkinson's, depression, migraines and scoliosis have a new approach in treatment.

To me, natural healing involves hygienic living (pure food, water, air, exercise, etc.), detoxification of metals, chemicals and toxins, treatment of infective organisms and optimization of structure. This is a paradigm shift in medicine.

Why aren't good diet, exercise and rest enough to correct all my health problems and to optimize my structure?

The body has emotional, mechanical and biochemical functions. The nature of your biochemical lifestyle does not make much difference to your mechanical operation. It is similar to a car. If you have an accident with your car, it can't function normally until you fix the body and chassis. Just replacing fuel filters and oil or adding gasoline will not repair the car after an accident. Thinking positive thoughts will not take the dents out of our cars or our bodies. We have had many accidents during our lifetimes. We also need the structural repairs. This is what NCR does.

Why does NCR help so many diverse conditions?

NCR is a technique that optimizes the function of the brain and body. It treats the cause of many conditions. If you have chronic pain in the musculoskeletal system, the pain can go away by optimizing the musculoskeletal system. If you have a problem with brain function, NCR can help by optimizing the mechanical function of the brain.

How do you know NCR works?

I have been a naturopathic physician since November of 1982. I performed thousands of treatments on thousands of patients. Throughout those years, I never saw the results nor got the positive patient feedback that I get from NCR. ***I am certain that NCR works because I can see the results every day.***

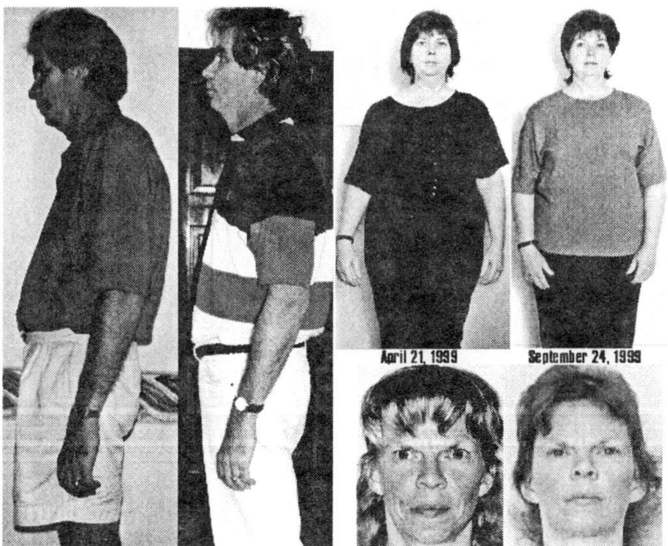

April 21, 1999 — September 24, 1999

September 8, 1997 — February 5, 1998 — August 19, 1996 — June 19, 1998

II. General Information

Can everyone benefit from NCR?

Yes. I have never seen a perfect skull and spine. This means that some amount of treatment could be useful for everybody, even though they may have no presenting complaints.

How many treatments do I need? Why do some people need more treatments than others do?

I never know how many treatments any person may need. This is for two reasons:

1) People have different reasons for seeking therapy—

For instance, some people seek NCR because of a specific pain or area of trouble in their bodies. For them, they will stop treatment as soon as their problem stops. When people have simple conditions like sinusitis, as few as four treatments may be all that is needed to stop the sinus problems. With other conditions, like dystonia or severe spinal problems, treatment could last 20 four-treatment sessions without exhausting the potential for continued improvement.

Other people have larger, less concrete goals when they receive therapy. If a person wishes to optimize their bodily functions (as I do) or they have serious or complicated conditions affecting their health, treatment can be more of an open-ended situation—they can get treatments for a long time.

Neither of these groups of people is right or wrong. Either of these plans can be right for the individual. Some people may even change their concepts as treatment progresses, and this is fine too. The nature of NCR treatment, with its essentially permanent results, allows a person to stop treatment at almost any time (after the completion of each treatment sequence).

2) Bodies change at different rates—

I have never known of two people who had identical bodies. This is because people have different genetic forms and different life experiences. By the time people come to me for treatment, they are unique, individual structures. In a way, people are like puzzles for me to untangle. Some puzzles are easier to solve than others, and some people's bodies change more quickly than others. I never know how fast a person will change. I never know how much a person will move from a single treatment. I never know what tomorrow's treatment will cause or require. I simply, continually release the obstructions in a person's structure that prevent him/her from moving towards the ideal structure the body was designed to have, free of deformity of life's traumas.

Do a lot of people return for further treatment?

Yes. Most people find it necessary to return for more than one treatment sequence to get the results they desire. For most, four or five treatment sequences (sixteen or twenty treatments) is a likely treatment requirement.

How long does each treatment take?

NCR is scheduled to last thirty minutes each day. This includes the time with the doctor and the NCR massage.

Why do you schedule treatments four days in a row? Is there a limit to how many treatments I should get in a row? How long should I wait between sequences?

Experience has taught me that isolated treatments are less effective than clusters of treatments. In a manner similar to getting momentum as you roll down a hill, the skull gains movement speed as treatments accumulate day after day. This means that results that cannot be created with isolated treatment become more predictable with dense treatment sequences. It is, however, more intense than getting treatments one at a time. Generally, after four days of treatment, a person is ready to rest from the rigors of NCR. With enthusiastic, NCR-experienced persons, I will permit more than four days of treatment in a row. My most extreme treatment situation, so far, has been thirty-two treatments in one month!

After four days of treatment, a person continues to change for three weeks or more. This is why I advise a person to wait for a period of time between treatment sequences. In unusual situations in which a person needs to have six or more treatments in than two weeks, I will have them wait for a longer period of time before they can resume normal, vigorous activities.

For patients who are interested in changing very rapidly, I recommend that they average four treatments monthly (one treatment sequence every four weeks). On the other end, there are some people who see me for a treatment sequence once annually, and they continue to show cumulative improvements. For the average person, having a treatment sequence every two to four months is a very satisfactory rate of change. At this treatment frequency, the speed of improvement is slow enough to prevent the flu and fever reactions that can be associated with rapid change.

Why do you take pictures before and after each series?

While NCR treatment accumulates, changes in the appearance of the face and the position of the spine, head and pelvis are constant. Nobody can remember that many details about a person's appearance. I continue to take photos after each treatment sequence to document these changes.

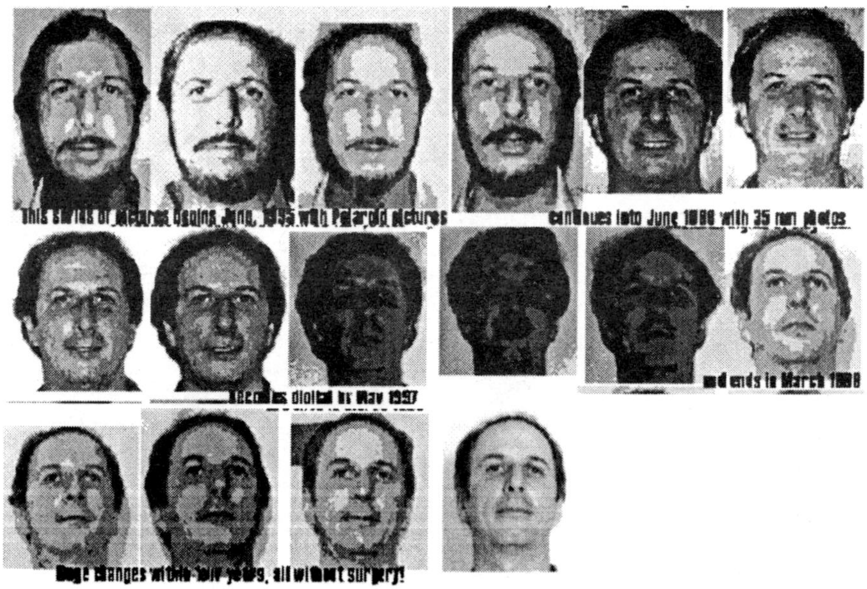

How long can I keep getting benefits from each treatment series and from NCR in general?

Each NCR treatment sequence is long lasting. Most of the changes are permanent. However, people's emotional life, the nature of their work/activities and the therapies they receive from dentists and others, is continually traumatizing most people. For these problems, most people find that they need to get more NCR sequences occasionally.

Additionally, there is no reason to stop receiving treatment; nobody is perfect. As long as the head, spine and pelvis are not perfect, there is room for more improvement in the structure and the mind with further treatment. For those people who wish to be their best, NCR is part of the path.

Consider those people who strive to become more perfect and develop psychic or spiritual abilities. How can they achieve these things with a brain that is not performing optimally? Of course it is important to perfect the lifestyle and the physical and mental activities of one's life, but without structural optimization, there will be a limitation on the amount of improvement available.

I predict that NCR will become an important facet in the developmental process for higher consciousness.

How long after having a fracture to my nose can I begin treatment? What are the precautions in treating me?

Without X-ray, many apparently broken noses are misdiagnosed. Many injuries are only displacements of the nasal bones. Endonasal balloons can be used to set a displaced or broken nose. This is often better than the common orthopedic techniques. With a true nasal fracture, after the bones are well set, NCR treatment should be delayed until the fracture is fully healed. In questionable cases, X-ray should confirm this. Generally six to twelve weeks is a sufficient waiting period.

What are the youngest and the oldest ages of people you can treat with NCR?

Babies need to be born before NCR can be begun, and the sooner they are treated the better. There is no upper limit for treatment, as long as the patient is still alive.

Will I feel okay to go out to eat after a treatment? What about eating before my treatment?

It is best to eat only lightly before treatment. Sometimes treatment can feel very powerful, and it is more comfortable not to be full at that time.

Your appetite should be just fine soon after treatment. After NCR you usually feel disoriented for about fifteen minutes. Less than twenty per cent of the people have long-lasting effects like fever, cold symptoms or headache after that. Just eat sensibly (as you always should)!

Do other doctors practice NCR?

Yes. Look at the NCR website at www.ndnd.com or contact my office at PO Box 448, Tonasket, WA 98855 and the list of NeuroCranial Restructuring Doctors' Association certified practitioners will be available.

Who is eligible to be trained as a NCR therapist? How long does the initial training take and what does it cost?

A doctor whose licensure permits endonasal therapy techniques could be accepted into my training program for NCR. Classes are limited to six doctors for an intense, one-week course. The class takes about sixty hours and costs $3000. The course includes four treatments from me, a set of before-and-after treatment photos of each participant, enough equipment to begin practicing NCR, observation of me performing at least forty treatments, observation of other doctors performing forty-five more treatments and personally treating two patients for four days while I supervise.

What's involved in my being a patient for a student doctor during one of the NCR training courses? How much does it cost to be seen by a student doctor?

When there is a training class, there are spaces available for up to twelve patients. These people are generally inexperienced with NeuroCranial Restructuring. The current charge for the training course is $250 for a four-treatment series, including an orientation talk from the training doctor, four treatments from the training doctor while I supervise and a set of before-and-after treatment photographs. Sign up for these spaces with my front office staff. My ability to accept training patients is conditional on having doctors sign up for a training class. Not all the dates set aside for training can be used for NCR courses.

Help me recruit doctors of good potential for the NCR training courses!

III. Anatomy, Structure and NCR

Why does my spine and whole nervous system shift from moving my head?

The main job of the spine is to hold the body upright. This is particularly true of the neck and upper back. Holding the head in a stable position is the job of the neck bones and muscles and is especially important because most of the nervous system is housed inside the head. An unstable skull means that the center of the nervous system is unstable too. The chronic positions of the spine and its related muscles are determined by the nervous system's need to maintain skull stability. When the positions of the bones of the skull are changed, the balancing pattern of the head is changed. This causes alterations in the postural patterns of the spine and the Para spinal muscles.

Nervous system functions are determined by the flow of blood and cerebrospinal fluid. When we use mood-altering drugs, they cause shifts in the flow of blood and especially cerebrospinal fluid, changing the amounts of neurotransmitters received by specific neurons (in the brain) and altering nervous system function. The shape of the skull and spine help determine the flow of blood and cerebrospinal fluid and thereby control nervous system function.

So when the shape of the skull is changed, the shape of the spine and pelvis are changed too, and through this the function of the nervous system is different as well. When the structural shape is improved (or even optimized) the nervous system functions are improved (optimized) too.

What causes my cranial bones to become unbalanced in the first place?

Your cranial bones are not unbalanced, but their asymmetrical structural alignment can cause difficulties for the function of the brain and nervous system as well as the musculoskeletal structure. The bones are in their stable, asymmetrical alignment pattern because of the body's reaction to the physical, biochemical and emotional traumas it has been subjected to. The most obvious, common traumatic events that most people experience are normal vaginal births. The intense squeezing of the head during birth, known as cranial molding, almost always leaves its mark on the adult skull. This affects both skeletal growth patterns and nervous system function for the life of the individual unless it is removed from the system. Similarly, falls, beatings, sports injuries, motor vehicle accidents, surgeries, dental work and the like all have long-lasting impact on the nervous system and musculoskeletal system.

How does moving my sphenoid move all the other cranial bones?

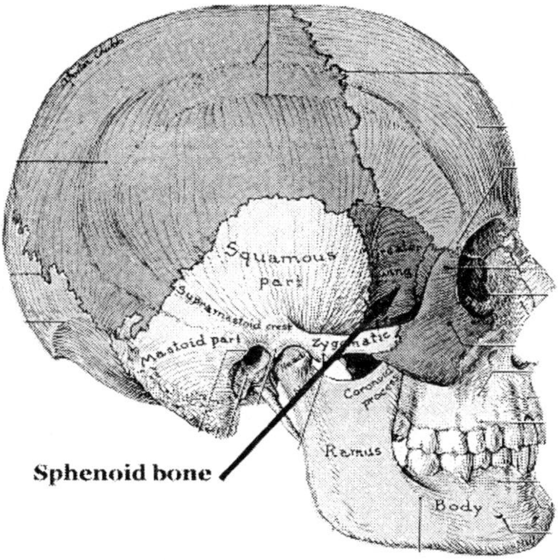

In the cranial structure, the sphenoid bone sits in the center. It is in contact with almost all the other bones of the skull, and they interlock. It is impossible to move any single bone of the skull without moving the bones adjoining it, eventually affecting them all. The sphenoid bone is the strongest, the most difficult to get manual contact with, the most difficult to move, the most resistant to change. Without moving the sphenoid bone, no other cranial bone movement can last. It is only by moving the sphenoid bone that all the bones of the head can be moved because of the sphenoid bone's central location. And it is only by moving the sphenoid bone in a pattern that is proprioceptively correct that the sphenoid bone can be moved in a lasting way.

How can my skull, which is made of bone, expand and contract?

Bone is not rigid when it is alive, having instead plasticity that allows a small amount of bending under stress. Additionally, when functioning properly, a skull will have some movement capability in all the joints of the skull. In an ideal head there are no truly fused joints, despite what you may read in old anatomy books. The bones of the head are in constant motion. Dr. Viola Fryman, D.O. proved this beyond a doubt in 1962 when she measured the motions of the skull during breathing and chewing with many small sensors place across the bones of the head.

How do my neurotransmitter levels change from receiving treatment?

Neurotransmitters, an essential part of nervous system functioning, are chemicals that allow nerves to send signals amongst themselves. These chemicals flow across the gap between adjacent nerves as well as circulating through the cerebrospinal fluid, allowing nerves, both close and distant, to communicate with one another.

Drugs used to treat depression, like Prozac and Elavil, work by changing the amount of a neurotransmitter, serotonin, throughout the nervous system. Researchers find that increased levels of serotonin decrease feelings of depression. The problems with antidepressant drugs are the side effects on most people, including decrease in sex drive, increase in anxiety and other symptoms that were previously not found in the patient. My clinical observation is that these patients had poor distribution of the neurotransmitter rather than deficiencies (lack of secretion) of serotonin. If the distribution problems in the nervous system were solved, the depression would decrease or stop.

When I treat depressed people with NCR, their depression gradually goes away. NCR optimizes the shape of the nervous system support structures, the bones of the skull and spine. With optimal shape, fluid flow characteristics of the blood and cerebrospinal fluid are idealized as well. The distribution of neurotransmitters gradually equalizes with NCR, becoming the distribution pattern we were designed to have instead of the distribution pattern our trauma histories have created. This is why I have good treatment results with depression, obsessive-compulsive disorder, seizures, learning disabilities, hyperactivity, Parkinson's disease, Alzheimer's disease and others. All of these conditions have significant structural problems in the skull contributing to the severity of the disease.

Can NCR prevent or reverse age-related stooping?

Yes. Even though the stooping posture is considered to be a consequence of osteoporosis, age-related stooping is actually a simple change in posture. As the posture worsens, there is also bone loss. This is because bone grows most strongly in areas where the gravitational force is greatest and does not grow where there is no gravitational force. When posture is poor, there is less weight carried by the bones, so the gravitational force in the bone is diminished, and the bone has fewer minerals secreted, leading to a lessening of its ability to support the body's weight (and increasing the weight that the musculature must support, leading to chronic muscular tension). This means that there is less stimulation of bone growth when posture is poor. With NCR, posture improves, forcing the bones to support more weight. Increasing the weight that the bones support stimulates more secretion of bone material and the bones grow stronger again.

Posture changes because most postural problems are created from the spine's difficulty in supporting the skull. As the head is positioned more forward on top of the neck, the head tips slightly forward and the body are pulled forward by the weight of the head, leading to a stooped posture. The role of NCR in this situation, then, is to change the position of the head relative to the neck, allowing a more balanced position of the head and greater ease of support by the neck. When this occurs, the spine is no longer in the poor posture.

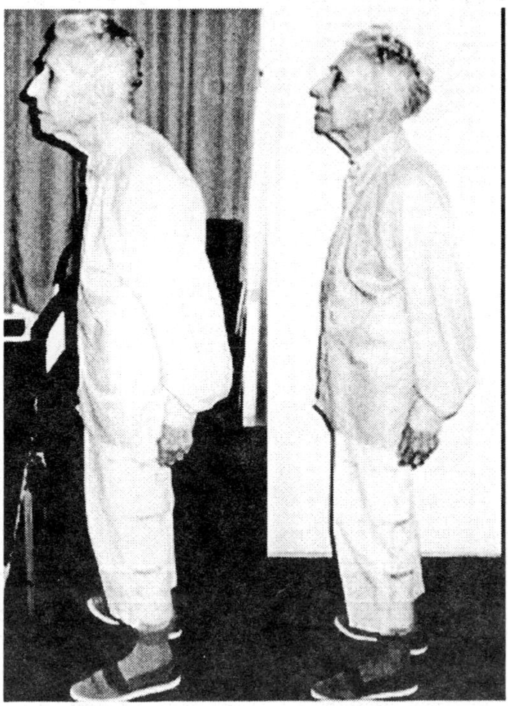

Before After

The brain is very sensitive to these balance patterns that create posture. The balance process is part of proprioception, a crucial part of the theories underlying NCR. The entire pattern of musculoskeletal posture is determined by proprioception—the awareness of the body's position in space, and the semicircular canals of the ears are an important part of this process. When the semicircular canals are stimulated frequently, the brain must work harder. The nervous system doesn't like this, and it responds by moving the musculoskeletal system into a position where less head movement occurs. This stable position of the head is known as our postural pattern. For many people, the postural pattern remains the same throughout their life. This is because the bones of the head are very stable, and these persons had no therapy or trauma that changes this cranial balancing pattern.

Your postural pattern is determined by your balance pattern. Subtle movements of the semicircular canals are very perceivable by the brain. The brain wishes to be stable, and will change the position of the spine and muscles to insure stable positioning of the skull. It is only by changing the shape of the skull that the body's balancing patterns can be changed, and in this way change the pattern of posture.

IV. NCR Technique

How do you diagnose how many balloons to use and where?

When I examine you, I am running *proprioceptive* tests. This is my way of determining which areas of your body are not under stable control by your balance system. The areas that are under good proprioceptive control should not be treated at the time. They should be left alone.

This is the problem that can be created by treating the area of the body that has pain. The stability of the body can be made worse so that the results of therapy will be merely temporary. It is only through treatment of the appropriate areas that predictable and cumulative results can be seen.

At this time, this can be accomplished only through great personal insight of the therapist (luck) or with proprioceptive testing. The tests are conducted in standing, seated and supine positions. When the testing is complete for the day, I have a picture of the binding forces or lock patterns of the connective tissues in the skull, spine and pelvis. Once I understand this, I know the position in which I need to place your pelvis, head and neck and which positions in the nose need balloons as well as the number and kinds of balloons.

The treatment unlocks the binding pattern in the skeletal system (rather like creating an earthquake), and the body begins shifting its pattern of stabilization.

What happens when the balloons are inflated?

The endonasal balloons are inserted through the nostril into the top of the throat through one of the six passageways that are available. The inflating bulb is squeezed, pumping air into the balloon, and it puffs up in the nostril. As the air pressure in the balloon becomes greater, it presses outward against the bones inside the nose and upper throat. Eventually the pressure becomes great enough that the balloon forces its way into the top of the throat. At that instant the bony joints of the head are opened for a moment, and the tensions stored in the connective tissues are released. The bone structures of the head now shift.

What does depth of balloons mean?

When proprioceptive testing is completed for the day, some of the findings include a skull map. The positions of the skull that I have found important for treatment can be generalized as anterior (shallow), intermediate or posterior (deep). This is important for the choice of the shape of the inflating balloons. To reach a deeper joint in the head, thicker balloons (greater gauge) are required. Shallower depths are reached with thinner balloons. These variations will make the treatment feel different to the patient at the moment of inflation, but the changes felt after inflation will not differ.

Why is there a special massage before the balloons?

NCR is a therapy technique that changes the entire structural system, including the bones and muscles. By using NCR massage techniques, the general muscular structure can be changed to allow a simpler skeletal alignment pattern. However, the massage alone is not sufficient to create long-lasting changes, because massage treats only the muscles, and the balance pattern of the bones is the final factor in determining the chronic muscle tension and postural patterns.

The release of the muscles from their typical tension also releases tension inside the skull, spine and pelvis. This temporarily brings the bony structures closer to their ideal position, although in a manner that is inherently unstable. (Without appropriate bone movement, these changes are only temporary.) This means that NCR balloon treatment can be more effective and more comfortable because there is less mechanical resistance to movement of the bones toward their ideal position.

Why do you place my body in a special position during treatment?

Inside the skull and connecting through the spinal column with the pelvis is the meningeal system. It is comprised primarily of very strong and long, elastic connective tissue fibers. Eighty-five per cent of the meninges are found inside the skull. The remaining fifteen per cent surround the spinal cord and connect to the pelvis. The specialized bodily positions used during NCR place additional stress on the meningeal fibers from the pelvis through the spine and into the skull. This allows a greater and more complete shift of the entire system at the time the balloon is inflated.

In the past, NCR therapy was combined with mild adjustments of the spine and pelvis. When appropriate bodily positions are included with the balloon treatment, no other manipulations are needed. In fact, the need to include the spinal and pelvis adjustments was an indication of incomplete cranial therapy of the musculoskeletal system!

Is there anything I can do to accelerate my progress with NCR?

Yes. Active movements, if within a person's normal performance range, are helpful, especially balanced activities like walking, yoga, ta'i chi or some kinds of swimming. It is important to stop exercising before much fatigue sets in.

If emotional tension and anxiety are prominent during a treatment series, then relaxant herbs and medications are very important.

If rapid progress is desired, treatment intervals should average less than twelve weeks but at least four weeks. This is the most efficient use of therapy. Some people, who lack the time for travel, are concentrating treatments into smaller time capsules and this works satisfactorily too. But these concentrated treatments create the potential for side effects from the changing structural patterns that are undetectable by the treating doctor that can lead to painful postural patterns, necessitating further treatment.

There has been a good treatment result with an experimental treatment protocol of twenty-four treatments in a month! In this situation, though, there was additional significant short-term side effects. There was great tenderness of the mucous membrane in the nose, and the following four to six weeks the patient's body was constantly changing, so he needed to be even more careful to avoid any traumatizing activities than any NeuroCranial Restructuring patient needs to be.

Is there anything that impedes my progress with NCR? What should I avoid?

Yes. Please avoid potentially traumatic activities and extremes in emotions or fatigue. Common daily activities can be harmful soon after receiving NCR treatment.

Any activity that stresses the muscles or bones in an unusual way can change the postural pattern, and before stability is achieved (after a treatment sequence) damage can occur. If you are not a furniture mover, don't begin moving furniture just after completing NCR. If you normally walk three miles daily, then walk three miles daily---don't decide to walk five miles because you're feeling so good.

If you're feeling good after receiving NCR, don't return to your therapist for massage or manipulation because it is your normal appointment time. (If their work were so great and effective, then you wouldn't have needed NCR.)

Massage, osseous manipulations, dental work, working or exercising to extreme limits, great fatigue or getting highly emotional can be detrimental to your NCR results. Please wait at least three weeks before beginning these sorts of activities. If you are still aware of movement going on, delay even longer. After stability is achieved, such activities will be no problem; there will be fewer difficulties in activity or mobility than there were before receiving the NCR.

V. NCR vs. Other Therapies

What makes NCR different from all other therapies?

NCR is the only physical medicine technique that routinely expects to produce permanent, cumulative changes to the skull, spine, pelvis and nervous system. Other physical medicine techniques require their patients to return for maintenance visits so that the effects of treatment can last. This is because other techniques are not including proprioceptive testing, which allows the NCR doctor to insure that the treatment is always improving the system's overall performance. When the system's stability is improved, there is no reason for the system to return to the older stability pattern. This allows treatments that are essentially permanent. No other treatment technique has these sorts of results predictably. For them, permanent results are the exceptional case, not the routine.

How is NCR different from craniosacral therapy?

Craniosacral therapy descends from the osteopathic cranial manipulation techniques begun by Dr. William Sutherland, D.O. and further modified and improved by Dr. John Upledger, D.O. Therapists performing craniosacral therapy use only their hands on the patient's head and mouth. They use pressures no greater than five grams (not quite enough pressure to squish a grape). Craniosacral therapy is designed to balance the distribution of cerebrospinal fluid.

NCR has a heritage less documented. It began with finger technique in the 1920s, which was improved to include the small endonasal balloons in the 1930s (then known as bilateral nasal specific technique), improved further by Dr. J. Richard Stober, D.C., N.D. in the 1960s and 1970s, who taught it to me from 1980 to 1984.

I developed the concepts of NCR in 1995, and the technique is being constantly modified and improved. The primary precept of NCR is to optimize nervous system and musculoskeletal functions by simplifying structure and improving structural stability. Like craniosacral therapy, NCR is very concerned with the flow of cerebrospinal fluid. With NCR, however, to change the skull, the major focus is movement of the sphenoid bone, which is poorly accomplished with the hands alone. To move the sphenoid, I find the endonasal balloons to be most effective. At this time, I have found that the sphenoid and related cranial bones can require more than twenty-five pounds of force to release the inflexible cranial joints.

So you can see that NCR and craniosacral therapies have some common concepts and goals, but our methods of evaluation and treatment have very little in common.

Can I have NCR in place of some dental work? How long after treatment should I wait to have dental work done? What is the proper protocol for dental work with NCR?

Most kinds of dental work will not be replaced with NCR. Unfortunately, your bridges, crowns, fillings or dentures will not be corrected by this treatment. But the work done by dentists specializing in TMJ, bite problems, dental orthopedics or orthodontia can often be avoided or simplified. Generally these dental techniques are trying to correct problems created by the skull shape by working on only part of the skull. This is not very efficient. If the work is begun with NCR, the need for local dental treatment is much reduced.

If you suspect that you require dental assistance with bridges, crowns, dentures, your tooth position or your bite, get NCR first, then get the dental work, return for some NCR and finish with some dental fine-tuning. If you are getting cosmetic bonding, cleaning, periodontal treatment or a basic filling, there is less concern unless you have a tendency towards TMJ, in which case the long sessions of holding your mouth open will cause changes in your head shape.

Please avoid getting dental diagnosis or therapies for at least a month after completing a sequence of NCR as your head and mouth will still be shifting during this time.

Why does my spine keep going back into a painful position after chiropractic adjustments and how is NCR different?

The shape of the head determines the position that the vertebrae need to be in to best support the head. This determines the spinal/pelvic posture. When local treatment of the spine is performed, the entire musculoskeletal system pattern, including the skull, is not changed. The musculoskeletal system is normally in a stable position. Local treatment of the spine usually causes systemic instability. The system reacts to this instability by returning to a stable pattern. Most of the time this means that the body returns the spine to the previous stable and painful position. NCR, when properly performed, continually moves the skull and spine into newer, less painful and yet still stable patterns. This allows the NCR patient to be able to stay in the new alignment pattern.

Is NCR more effective cosmetically than plastic surgery?

NCR moves the bones of the skull to the position where they were originally intended to be. This means that the skin will now fit properly, with the lines and wrinkles that appear in later life dramatically decreased, the nose and eyes straighter and more even and the jaw more centered, with no annoying TMJ click. This removes the need for plastic surgery, which is simply a technique for reworking the bones and (especially) the skin to positions where the skin looks tight. NCR is more effective than cosmetic surgery because the asymmetry found in most faces can be corrected. Eyes that appear to be different shapes, a crooked mouth, uneven cheekbones, ears that don't line up—all of these are always improved with NCR. Besides looking better with NCR, a patient feels and functions better too.

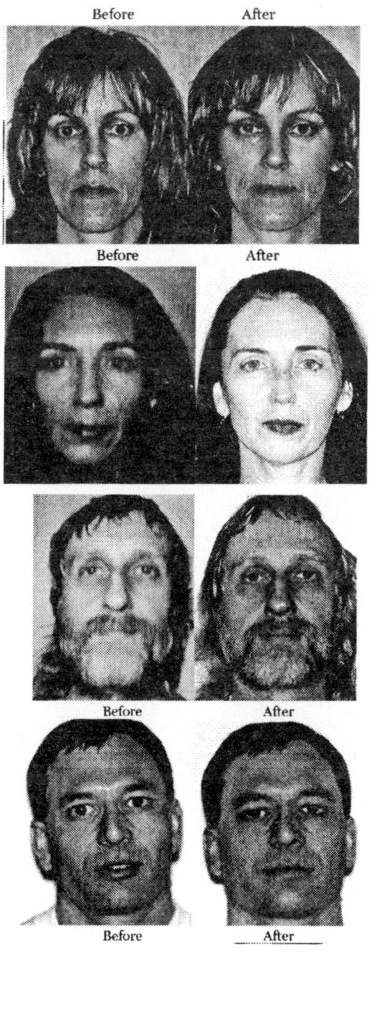

VI. Effects and Results of NCR

Does treatment hurt?

Everyone notices intense pressure inside the nose during each treatment with the endonasal balloons. The pressure is used one or two times daily for two to five seconds each time. This means that each treatment has from two to twenty seconds of intense pressure inside the nose. Treatment sometimes hurts. Some people find the first treatment sequence very painful. Each day, after treatment, the bones continue to move, and this too can feel strange, painful or uncomfortable. These situations are usually most intense during the first treatment series. Fortunately, it doesn't remain that way. Ninety-five percent of the return patients find it easier after the first sequence.

Can I function normally right after a treatment?

No. After NCR treatment, a person needs to rest for (typically) five to fifteen minutes before driving. Occasionally a longer time is needed for recuperation. After this initial reaction time, normal tasks like driving can be performed. However, people can have residual effects, such as sensations of movement in the head (aching or throbbing), cold or flu symptoms, or increased fatigue, so that they may not feel like they are functioning normally for the entire treatment series and a few days beyond.

Might I vomit or have a toxic release after treatment?

I have performed about sixty thousand treatments with endonasal balloons. I have seen two or three episodes of vomiting. It is so rare that I do not think these cases were associated with treatment.

However, it is reasonably common to have toxic releases after NCR. During early treatment series, as many as one of six patients can have detoxification reactions like fever, diarrhea or malaise.

What should I do if I easily bleed, bruise or am on blood thinners?

If you bleed easily, be prepared for the possibility of blood during NCR treatment. I have only seen visible bruising with endonasal balloons twice, and the last case occurred more than fifteen years ago. For internal bruising, I recommend the enzyme bromelain (from pineapple) as well as the homeopathic *Arnica montana* to promote healing. Using blood thinners is usually no problem. In special circumstances, with the permission of the prescribing doctor, some patients will decrease their blood thinner dosage for a few days prior to NCR.

What if I have a tendency to blackout?

It is common to feel light-headed after NCR treatment. Homeopathic medicines such as *Arnica* or *Gelsemium* are usually effective in stopping this quickly. But, very rarely, people have fainted. All NCR staff members try to prevent blackout by not standing you up too quickly and by letting you sit or lie down when you feel faint. The feeling will pass soon.

How does NCR affect pregnant and delivering women? Are there any precautions?

NCR is not recommended during labor and delivery. There are too many other things for the mother to be concerned with at that time. However, treatment can be given at any time up to that point. It is best to work on a pregnant mother early in her pregnancy because she will be more comfortable throughout the pregnancy and delivery when her spine and pelvis are operating optimally. If the treating doctor finds that a pregnant woman has powerful changes during NCR treatment, then therapy should be avoided during the final trimester of pregnancy so that labor isn't begun prematurely. (I know of no instance of this occurring.)

How does NCR affect athletic performance?

NCR is one of the most innovative ways of improving athletic performance. Many athletes strive for perfect form with bodies that work imperfectly. For instance, when a sprinter runs, the arms should be pumped straight forward and back. This can occur only if the shoulders are in the correct anatomical position. If the postural pattern of the athlete is not optimal, he or she cannot run as fast because of the inability to pump the arms efficiently and effectively. This is one of many such situations that can be corrected with NCR.

Many athletes now wear nasal breathing tapes to open the nasal passages. But with NCR, nasal breathing can be greatly improved without the need for tapes across the nose.

Remember the 1998 Super Bowl in which the running back for the Denver Broncos needed a drug injection during halftime to control his migraine pain? Orthodontia had decreased the severity of his migraines, and he had the best season of his athletic career. With a hit to his head during the first quarter of the Super Bowl, a migraine appeared. With NCR, his migraines could be stopped.

Many athletes cannot run as fast or as far as they would like because of the inability to breathe deeply. This is especially true when the excursion of the diaphragm is reduced. With NCR, the musculoskeletal structures are released and diaphragm movement is enhanced, creating a larger, deeper breath every inhalation. This allows the more efficient aerobic respiration to continue longer in the body, delaying the inevitable anaerobic respiration. This means the athlete can run longer, farther and faster before fatigue sets in.

NCR for athletes is a natural solution for athletic enhancement!

How long does my head keep shifting after treatment?

Typical head movement lasts for three weeks after treatment. In unusual situations, people have felt continued movement in their heads for four months.

What happens if I keep getting treatments after my symptoms disappear? What does NCR do besides relieving conditions and their symptoms? Can I grow as a person from NCR? How?

As NCR treatments continue, the benefits accumulate. The body continues to move closer and closer to its original blueprint. This means that the benefits become more profound as treatment continues. At first, symptoms of pain and obvious dysfunction leave. Later other beneficial changes are experienced as the nervous system and musculoskeletal systems optimize. This is the time when people note profound transformations in their personalities and in the way they think, feel and move.

The brain develops the feelings a person has. The concept of separation of the mind and body, developed by Descartes in the seventeenth century, is not real. If this were so, ingesting drugs could not alter mental state. This is why counseling is used only for minor psychiatric maladies, and the severe psychiatric states are treated with drugs. With a severe psychiatric state, the brain does not work right! This is not a situation a person can be talked out of. This is also why tense, anxious people look forward to a cup of tea or a glass of wine or beer after a hard day. Do you know anyone who needs coffee in the morning to lift his or her morning depression? All of these examples are indications that the mind is a part of the brain/body.

Although it sounds more spiritual to keep it separate, in reality the spirit is housed in the body/mind. So changing mental function makes a person different in ways a person cannot comprehend without experiencing it him or herself. This can be accomplished through life experiences, both good and bad, both traumatic and euphoric, and created dependably through changing the shape of the head with NCR.

There is a growing cadre of people who continue receiving NCR treatments because of the personal growth they are achieving. Only a body that is operating nearly perfectly can achieve true spiritual growth, the sort that people dream about. How, for instance, can a person expect an imperfectly operating brain to develop psychic skills or achieve a state of peace and bliss? A necessary prerequisite is to optimize brain function. When there is idealized flow of blood and cerebrospinal fluid, brain functioning can be optimal, if the other criteria are met. But a person seeking to become more perfect (by perfecting diet, physical, mental and emotional activities) who does not optimize the mechanical function of the skull can never achieve optimal function of the brain and body.

Does NCR have any bad side effects?

The bad side effects of NCR are all short term. Typical reactions that may occur after treatment include light-headedness, headache, runny and stuffy nose, fever, nosebleed, tearfulness and flashbacks of past events.

The only bad long-term effect is the possible temporary reoccurrence of pain symptoms. Even though this is unpleasant, this is not a bad sign for the body. It is just a movement of the skeleton that is parallel to a position that the body had in the past. With continued treatment, these situations have always reversed.

What are some good NCR side effects?

Many people seek NCR treatment because of a specific complaint, like headaches, sleep apnea or back pain. But NCR cannot be focused towards a specific complaint but is instead a generalized treatment that corrects the causes of many symptoms. People report that they feel more energetic, happy, athletic, clear-headed, smart, creative and (of course) beautiful. After undergoing NCR, people have better nasal breathing, smoother action of the TMJ, better posture, improved vision, better balance, decreased muscle tension, decreased emotional tension and less pain.

Why do I feel clearer, calmer and happier after receiving NCR treatment?

The feelings of clearness, calmness and happiness are part of the normal state of the mind. People should always feel this way. When structures of the skull are not in their ideal positions, mechanical tension is found in the meningeal tissues. The brain has subtle pressures exerted on it by the malpositioned bones. These tensions and poor bone alignments cause the emotions perceived by the nervous system to be less than ideal. A person may feel grouchy, confused, anxious or other undesirable feelings. When the structures are optimized and the mechanical tensions are released, the functions of the nervous system are improved, and the normal emotional states ensue.

Why does my face change shape with treatment? Why does it tend to become more oval and symmetrical?

NCR is a method of optimizing (or simplifying) bodily structures. With it we remove the mechanical changes that trauma has inflicted on the body. As treatment progresses, the bones move closer and closer to the alignment pattern they were designed and formed to be in. For most people this means that their faces become more oval. For everyone, the structures become more symmetrical.

Before After

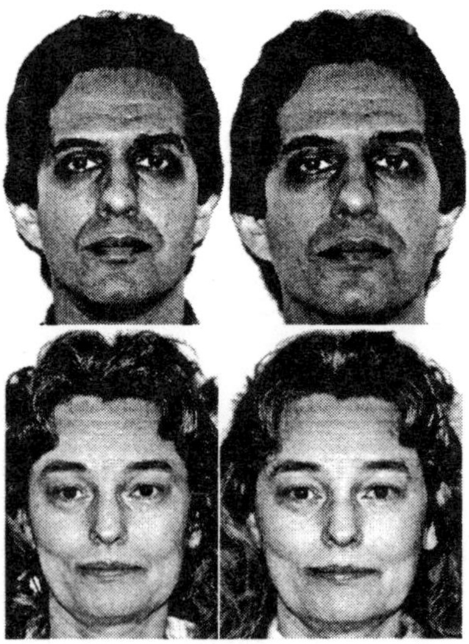

How do vitamins and minerals flow after treatment? Might I need to change my supplement dosages? Why?

Vitamin and mineral levels will not change from NCR treatment. However, because of the changes in nervous system functions, your supplement dosage levels may need to be different from before NCR. Remember that the utilization of all nutrients in the body is governed by the nervous system. Anything that changes functioning of the nervous system will change the body's requirements for nutrients.

What do I do if I get a strange reaction between sequences?

It is rare to have strange or uncomfortable reactions between sequences. When you do have these occur, it is an indication that your system has continued to move and change, and your structural state now requires further treatment. Unless you have an NCR-trained doctor or massage therapist available, you should see nobody else.

Why does my nose sometimes run or bleed after getting treatment?

It is very common to get a runny nose after NCR. There are two reasons for this: The sinuses are squeezed, causing them to dump their contents (of mucus), and the irritation of the mucous membranes of the nose cause watering of the eyes and increased manufacture of watery mucus. This reaction usually stops within two hours. Many people with chronic sinus problems look forward to a runny nose because this is a way to decrease their sinus pressure.

Nosebleeds can occur anytime the mucous membranes inside the nose are split or torn. This is especially common (about one of four patients) during the first treatment series of NCR when the skull structure is very tight. The movement of the skull at this time is more sudden (or brittle) than normal, and the mucous membranes split rather than stretch when the balloon inflates. As treatment continues, there is more elasticity in the skull structures, so that the mucous membranes have a chance to stretch rather than tear. Then bleeding does not occur.

Persons who have a history of nosebleeds find that the frequency and intensity of their nosebleeds diminish or stop after some NCR.

Why do my teeth sometimes ache after treatment?

The teeth are mounted in the bones of the head. NCR treatment releases the joints of the head so that the stored-up mechanical tension in the connective tissues of the skull, spine and pelvis (meninges, etc.) can be released. This release of tension is especially felt as movement of the bones of the skull. As the palate and jaw shift, the teeth move too. This can make the teeth ache, pulsate or tingle.

Why do my feet and arches look different after treatment?

The feet (and their arches) hold up the body. With NCR, as the structures begin to optimize, the weight distribution patterns of the body change. With this simplification of structure, the job of the feet (holding the body up) becomes easier. Less complicated foot shapes are required. The feet change shape, then, because of the change in their functional requirements.

VII. NCR Answers to Conditions

What is the protocol for comatose patients?

Comatose patients are treated like any others except proprioceptive testing cannot be performed in the sitting or standing positions. Please remember that the areas of the brain destroyed from the swelling and crushing during the closed-head injury will not be healed with NCR. However, the areas of the brain that are still viable and lack good circulation of blood and cerebrospinal fluid can have normal function restored with NCR.

Why does NCR treatment--which is structural--seem to help some of my biochemical problems such as poor digestion and post-nasal drip?

The nervous system controls all functions in the body, including digestion and manufacturing of mucus. Most of the nervous system is found inside the skull. With NCR, while the structures become more idealized, the nervous system functions are enhanced and many bodily processes normalize. This is why a wide variety of seemingly unrelated conditions can all improve with NCR.

How and why does NCR help the following conditions?

Alzheimer's?

Alzheimer's disease is associated with poor functioning of the brain. In autopsies Alzheimer brain tissue is dramatically different from regular brain tissue. A person suffering from Alzheimer's disease is not yet at the point of death, so their condition is somewhere between a normal person and death. Brain function is dependent on at least three factors: the state of the brain tissue, the flow characteristics of the blood and tissue, and the flow characteristics of the cerebrospinal fluid. Without the flow of blood and cerebrospinal fluid, the brain cannot function at all. Yet most therapeutic plans to treat Alzheimer's disease have focused on the brain tissue. This is why there are attempts to formulate new drugs as well as natural approaches using diet, detoxification of toxins and heavy metals, nutraceutical supplements and homeopathic medicines. These can help. But it is also important to insure that the fluid flow characteristics of the brain are optimized. This is where NCR can help. By improving the shape of the head, fluid flow patterns of the blood and cerebrospinal fluid can be improved, allowing the brain tissue to function at the peak of its capabilities. Granted, with

Alzheimer's disease, this will still be sub-optimal performance, but it will be a distinct improvement over the non-treated patient.

I have seen great results clinically, generally expecting to reverse two or three years of Alzheimer's symptoms in each four-day sequence. My doctor-students have had similar results. One doctor told me of an Alzheimer's patient whom her husband brought in. She received four days of NCR therapy, and each day had no memory of the previous day's treatment. Afterwards, her husband was delighted with her improvement, so he brought her back for more treatment three months later. When the doctor and her husband put her on the table she *remembered the treatment after three months.* She said, "No way you're going to do that to me again!"

NCR is an important part of a treatment protocol for Alzheimer's patients.

Anxiety and nervousness?

Anxiety is a condition of the brain. Drugs like Xanax and herbs such as kava kava, skullcap, valerian and hops have all been used successfully to treat anxiety symptoms. Sometimes counseling is effective for treatment of anxiety, but the patients who seek my care have found it ineffective. For them, the underlying cause of anxiety is a functional problem of the brain, so its treatment must address brain functioning.

Standard treatment techniques incorporate methods to change the levels of neurotransmitters in the brain. In this way, the areas of the brain that lack enough or have too much neurotransmitter can be normalized, temporarily alleviating the problem. The drugs and herbs used to treat anxiety temporarily change the levels of neurotransmitters in the brain. When the levels of neurotransmitters in the brain are raised or lowered, changes in feelings and behavior are seen and felt everywhere in the brain. This can often help a patient to feel less anxious.

The problem with medications is their lack of specificity in the brain. They make their changes throughout the brain instead of the specific area of the brain under concern. This can lead to side effects. The areas of the brain that have abnormal neurotransmitter levels (too high or too low) will change, hopefully in the way the doctor wishes. But the areas of the brain that already had normal levels of the neurotransmitter will now have the wrong level, leading to a side effect associated with the previously normal area of the brain now being over- or under-stimulated.

The problem of anxiety is associated with neurotransmitter levels. However, it is rarely a simple situation of under- or over-production but instead a problem of the distribution of neurotransmitters in the brain. Some areas of the brain have too low a level of some neurotransmitters, or some areas of the brain have too many neurotransmitters, or both situations are occurring simultaneously in different areas of the brain. This situation makes it difficult to give medications that are effective and without side effects.

The flow of cerebrospinal fluid and the flow of blood govern the distribution of neurotransmitters. The shape of the skull determines this. With NCR, the skull shape changes, altering the patterns of the flow of cerebrospinal fluid and blood. As the fluid flow characteristics change, the patterns of distribution of neurotransmitters are changed as well. The problem of the medications is circumvented with NCR. With NCR the distribution patterns of blood and cerebrospinal fluid can be normalized, ensuring normal levels of neurotransmitters throughout the brain.

As skull shape is optimized, then, the functioning of the brain becomes more optimal too. This creates a lasting change in conditions like anxiety.

Arthritis, bursitis and rheumatism?

Arthritis and rheumatism are conditions of the joints. NCR can change joint function in two major ways: through its ability to change:

1) the positions of the bones of the spine and pelvis, and
2) the nervous system.

People who have these conditions never have perfect posture. As NCR changes the postural patterns, the areas of pain and discomfort in the spine and pelvis diminish. When the weight-bearing patterns of the spine and pelvis are changed, the weight-bearing patterns of the hips, knees and feet change too. The sore points in the knee (for instance) will no longer be at the point of maximum weight bearing. This means that the position of the feet during walking (toe-in or toe-out, for instance) will not be the same. This can make incredible changes in a person's pain pattern.

The nervous system controls everything in the body, including the immune system. With conditions like rheumatoid arthritis or other autoimmune arthritides, optimizing immune function can make a great change in levels of inflammation.

I have rarely seen people with bursitis, yet I have seen many people wrongly diagnosed with bursitis. Fortunately, with these shoulder conditions, there is hope. Often the problem with a chronically frozen shoulder or other painful shoulder conditions is both postural and muscular. The muscular problems are often caused by the joint dysfunction created from the postural pattern, which triggers chronic spasms of the muscles to guard the body from performing painful joint movements.

This occurs especially after whiplash injuries, when the straightening of the neck and upper back (from the head moving too far forward from the injury) leads to a posture in which the shoulders are rolled forward and inward, accompanied by chronic muscle spasm of the neck, upper back and shoulders. When the shoulders are like this, performing normal shoulder activities like reaching toward the ceiling or combing the hair becomes mechanically impossible. A person cannot reach toward the ceiling if the shoulder joint is aimed at the wall and the muscles are as tight as cables. With NCR treatment, the postural pattern can be improved so that the shoulder is positioned more normally, allowing a person to return to more everyday activities.

Attention Deficit Hyperactivity Disorder, dyslexia and other learning disabilities?

Learning disabilities are frequently treated with prescriptions of Ritalin, a nervous system stimulant. The prevailing theory is that neurotransmitter deficiency in the brain leads to malfunctioning of the brain. The immediate solution is to increase neurotransmitter levels throughout the brain with Ritalin to correct the deficiency. This medication often helps, but it does not cure. It increases the levels of some neurotransmitters throughout the brain.

The effectiveness of Ritalin shows that learning disabilities are not psychological but are, instead, conditions created by problems with nervous system function. A nervous system stimulant like Ritalin works by changing levels of neurotransmitters in the cerebrospinal fluid in the brain. This means that inappropriate levels of neurotransmitters in specialized areas of the brain cause learning disabilities. When the brain lacks neurotransmitters in some areas, concentration or interpretation of visual or auditory phenomena is impaired. So increasing the level of these neurotransmitters helps to temporarily get rid of the problem.

Then why doesn't everybody with learning disabilities take Ritalin or some similar medication? The problem with administration of Ritalin is the side effects, which are generally symptoms associated with other areas of the brain becoming overdosed with neurotransmitters. If some areas of the brain improve function by increasing levels of neurotransmitters, and if other areas of the brain get side effects by increasing the same, there is a problem of distribution, not a deficiency of neurotransmitters. So the symptomatic treatment of learning disabilities with medication that increases the level of neurotransmitters can never cure the problem because it doesn't address the situation properly.

A cure of learning disabilities must include optimization of fluid flow characteristics in the brain. With optimal flow of blood and cerebrospinal fluid, learning disabilities improve or cease.

The approach of NCR is to improve the flow of cerebrospinal fluid (CSF) by changing the shape of the skull. As the cranium optimizes, the flow of CSF becomes more and more uniform, removing the problem of poor distribution of the fluids in the brain.

This seems like such a simple solution to an aggravating problem, and it is. But clinically it provides better results than the medications. There must be more truth to this model than the Ritalin deficiency model outlined above. Trust results!

Autism?

Autism is not understood and there is no predictable, effective treatment. I have worked with a few autistic children, and they have all been unique. But I think they all have problems with brain function, similar to those discussed with ADHD and hyperactivity. With autism, there is no simplified model that allows medications to control the symptoms. People who come out of their autistic state can shed little light on the cause(s) of autism. There are behavior control techniques that are opposed by some as being too harsh, but they are sometimes effective.

I have seen improvement in the autistic patients I have treated, but I find it slower and less predictable than with learning disabilities. Nonetheless, I believe that an important part of effective treatment of autism is to optimize the structures of the head and spine.

Brain surgery?

After brain surgery, NCR is very important.

The brain is surrounded by connective tissue, such as the meninges, and then by bone. This network of bone and connective tissue is interlocked and integrated. When they are changed, there are great implications for the functioning of the brain and body. The structures of the head are changed dramatically with surgery, and there are usually no efforts to return the head to its normal mechanical function.

After brain surgery, many people feel different from before. One woman I treated said that she was “fifty-seven going on ninety-seven”. Walking was difficult and painful. Her doctors had told her that she had little hope of improvement and prescribed medications to control her pain and inflammation. She felt old, stupid, tired and useless. The area of her skull that underwent surgery looked indented and rumpled. After receiving NCR treatment for three days, she performed high kicks for me and exclaimed, “I love you!” By this time, her surgical scars didn’t look the same anymore. Her skull was less depressed, and the skin was pulled more smoothly over the scar. As her skull had returned to a normal shape, her brain and body structures began working again the way they were designed.

Cerebral palsy?

Cranial therapy has been used for many years to treat persons with cerebral palsy. This is a condition with which my mentor, Dr. J. R. Stober, had dependable results using the old BNS therapy. NCR works even better. People whom I have seen with this condition generally fall into two classes: those with excessive muscle tone (they used to be called spastics) and those with too little muscle tone (we used to call this flaccid paralysis).

Both of these conditions are related to the level of functioning of the cerebellum, a part of the brain that controls muscle tone and the ability to stop movement once it has begun. One group has a hyper-functioning cerebellum and the other a hypo-functioning one. With NCR, once movement of the back of the head has been accomplished, the function of the cerebellum can be optimized. I know of no other therapy than NCR that can change the general condition of people with cerebral palsy.

Bipolar disorder (Manic-depression)? Depression? Obsessive-compulsive disorder? Psychosis? Schizophrenia?

Psychiatric conditions like depression, obsessive-compulsive disorder (OCD), schizophrenia, manic-depression and psychosis are rarely effectively treated with counseling. Most of the time, psychiatric drugs are prescribed. The common natural approaches are to mimic the effects of the drugs with less toxic substances that are similarly designed to change the levels of brain neurotransmitters. There are abnormalities (deficiencies) in the levels of neurotransmitters of the brain in the psychiatric-chemical model used to describe these treatment techniques. The drugs raise the level of the target neurotransmitter throughout the brain. This allows the areas of the brain previously deficient in the target neurotransmitter to have sufficient levels of neurotransmitter. The psychiatric condition is often controlled in this manner.

In the rare situation of a true neurotransmitter deficiency state, these medications perform brilliantly. They address the cause of the situation, the lack of neurotransmitter manufacture.

But most people on such medications experience side effects. Often the side effects are involved with functions that are not related to the actual complaint. A depressed person taking Prozac, for instance, can feel less depressed and have sexual impotence from the medication. These are problems of over-dosing the brain with the target neurotransmitter in the areas that had sufficient supply previously.

When one area of the brain has enough neurotransmitter and another area of the brain has too little or too much, this is not a problem of manufacture. It is a problem with uneven distribution of neurotransmitters.

The chemicals of the brain flow in liquid—blood and cerebrospinal fluid. The flow of fluid is determined partially by the shape of the vessel. The brain resembles a sponge in ways. A round sponge can be put into a cubical container, but it won't hold as much water in the areas that are squished to fit in the box. Likewise, a brain will not hold normal amounts of fluids when it is in an imperfectly shaped box.

With NCR, the shape of the skull gradually moves closer and closer to its optimal design. As the skull optimizes, the fluid flow characteristics of the skull, and the brain functions that are controlled by the fluid dynamics, optimize as well.

I have had clinical success with depression, obsessive-compulsive disorder (OCD) and bipolar disorder. The schizophrenics and psychotics I have worked with have been too suspicious of me to get enough treatment to receive any major benefits.

Concussion and other head injuries?

A concussion is a brain injury that results in a temporary loss of consciousness. This does not imply that there is significant, long-term damage to the brain. Concussion and other head injuries are the product of trauma. The normal medical procedure is to use X-rays or CAT scans to diagnose skull fractures and then watch to see if there is any indication of cerebral hemorrhage. Beyond that, there is no medical treatment. However, even with no measurable brain damage, there are long-term problems caused by concussions, and people should receive treatment for them.

The head trauma involves some sort of blow or fall on the head, and the cranial bones must be moved by it. This upsets the normal structural pattern that exists between the interlocking bones of the head, and it is unlikely or impossible for the head to resume its original position without treatment. This is a wonderful time to use NCR. I have treated many people after concussions, sometimes years later. The improvement that they experience is remarkable *and routine.* An NCR doctor should be on call in every hospital emergency room to treat all head injuries that do not have fractures or cerebral hemorrhage.

Down's Syndrome?

These people have a number of skull-related problems: poor vision, recurrent infections of the sinuses and middle ear, chronic nasal breathing difficulties, poor balance and posture, difficult speech, poor thinking and headaches.

Down's syndrome is very treatable with NCR. Dr. Stober, my mentor in endonasal therapy, specialized in treatment of Down's Syndrome individuals. Even with the old cranial therapies, they had dramatic improvement. As their nervous system functioning optimizes, improvements in speech, balance, vision and coordination are obvious. They seem smarter as well.

For example, my patient April [see testimonial] is now a high functioning Down's syndrome girl. She speaks intelligibly, walks normally and can ski the entire length of a mountain at her ski area.

Her eyes are losing their characteristic slant. She now has developed a nasal bridge and can breathe freely through her nose.

They are helped greatly with NCR.

Dystonia?

Dystonia is a condition affecting the brain stem—a part of the brain found low in the back of the head. Symptoms include blepharospasm, uncontrollable closing of the eyes, chronic and uncontrollable closure of the mouth, spasms of the muscles of the anterior throat, muscle tension headaches and uncontrollable writhing movements of the head/neck. There is no medical cure or even understanding of where the condition comes from. Medical therapy revolves around two treatments: 1) injections of botulism toxin to temporarily alleviate the annoyingly recurrent, uncontrollable muscle spasms and 2) prescriptions of tranquilizers and sedatives to calm these anxious, upset people.

I have worked with only five persons with dystonia and with only one for more than three treatment sequences. She is almost symptom free and has resumed her normal life. She no longer lives the life of a recluse, shunned by her family because of the stigma of a disease that distorts the person's appearance. It has taken thirty-six treatments (nine treatment clusters) to get her this far.

The other patients have had varying degrees of success. I believe that further treatment would give them lasting results. One lady who suffers from blepharospasm has short-term cessation of her symptoms. I think it would last longer with more treatment.

I hope to work with more cases of dystonia.

Ear infection (acute and chronic otitis media) and deafness?

Ear conditions have been treated for many years with endonasal therapy techniques with varying degrees of success. The ears are mounted within the temporal bones. The auditory nerve goes through the temporal bone on its way into the brain, and the Eustachian tubes, the passageways that connect the middle ears with the throat, are found between and through the temporal bones and the sphenoid.

When a person undergoes NCR treatment, the bones of the head gradually move into more optimal positions. This means that the position of the auditory nerve gradually moves into a more ideal location over time, and the drainage of the Eustachian tube becomes better and better.

This has immediate impact on acute and chronic ear infection (otitis media). When the Eustachian tubes are able to drain, the infection has no ability to develop pressure in the middle ear.

When I was in family practice, treating children with otitis media seemed to involve treatment of two causes—mechanical pressure of the bones against the Eustachian tubes and lymphatic pressure against the Eustachian tubes from infection or allergy. The use of antibiotics, whether synthetic or natural, was not effective. There are homeopathic medicines, botanical eardrops and hydrotherapy techniques that I used for acute treatment. In recurrent cases I employed the long-term approach, which was to change the diet and lifestyle and to perform NCR, which worked about ninety per cent of the time.

Deafness is a condition with multiple causes, some of them mechanical in origin, which are amenable to treatment with NCR. Overall, the people who experience improvement in their hearing have hearing loss from two causes:

1) Impingement of the auditory nerve, and
2) Chronic mucous congestion of the middle ear and Eustachian tube.

Many middle aged and senior adults have improvement in their hearing after receiving NCR, except those who lost their hearing from exposure to loud sounds. Many of these individuals have congestion of the Eustachian tubes (termed catarrhal deafness by old medical books).

NCR therapy changes the relative positions of the bones, resulting in better drainage of the middle ear. This decreases the pressure of the mucus against the eardrum, resulting in greater sensitivity of hearing. I have also worked with a few people who were born with ninety per cent or more hearing loss, and some of them have improvement with their hearing as well, although the improvement is still slight compared to their disability.

Forty-seven chromosome individuals?

I have never treated a patient of any age with Klinefelter's XXY. I have read the medical literature, and I think that NCR could be a wonderful treatment for this condition. Obviously, it will not repair the abnormal chromosomes, but it could help nonetheless by improving the overall state of nervous system functioning.

Glaucoma? Double vision? Other vision problems?

Glaucoma, an increase in the pressure inside the eyeball, is generally controlled with toxic medicated eye drops. The fear is that blindness will occur if the pressure in the eye gets too high. Every case of glaucoma I have treated in the past five years has improved enough that people either decreased or discontinued their glaucoma medication. I assume that the improvement in eye pressure occurs from movement of the sphenoid, frontal and maxillary bones that make up the eye socket. The movement of the bones into a more optimal position allows the fluid pressure in the eye to be relieved before the pressure gets too high.

Double vision is a condition in which the person is unable to focus their eyes without tremendous strain. Their comfortable eye position causes them to see two disparate images, hence the name double vision. The ability of the eyes to focus on a single image depends on the muscles of the eye working together. Double vision occurs when the eyes are unable to aim the visual field at the same image at the same time. When the images cannot superimpose, double vision results. There is no medical treatment of double vision besides prism installation in the glasses (to bend the visual image into an alignment in which the double vision is improved) or surgery for people who have one eye turned in or out.

The muscles of the eye work together in a simple fashion: they have common enervation. The brain sends out one signal, and matching muscles in each eye receive the signal. The muscles contract the same amount (because there is only one muscle contraction command), and normally the eyes move the same distance in the desired direction. But with asymmetrical eye sockets, the eyes move different distances with the same amount of muscle contraction. This makes visual focusing problematic and, in severe situations, it leads to double vision. NCR technique addresses this problem by changing the shapes of the orbits of the eyes. As the skull is optimized, the orbits of the eyes achieve their ideal shapes, and the visual focusing mechanism operates as it was designed.

I have had excellent results treating double vision with NCR. In severe cases, though, it could require twenty or thirty treatments to resolve.

Many people with visual problems like near- and far-sightedness will report improvement in their vision with NCR. Athletes report that they are able to see moving objects more clearly. I assume that this is because of the same mechanism I just described for double vision.

Headaches, head pressure and migraines?

Headache, head pressure and migraines are treated very successfully with NCR. Be sure to read the patient testimonials later in this book or at the NCR website http://www.ndnd.com. Headaches, head pressure and migraines have many causes such as head trauma, sinus infections, allergic sinusitis, constipation, TMJ, fever, colds, influenza, stress, eyestrain, glaucoma, hangovers and poisoning.

Of course, if you have a fever or poisoning, the biochemical and detoxification approaches used in naturopathic medicine are the obvious choices in treatment. Sometimes a simple liver flush, an enema and/or colonic irrigation or a short juice fast is good treatment for headaches, head pressure or migraines. But much of the time, these things are not enough.

The head encases the brain and meninges. The spine holds up the head, and its first bone (C-1) is known as the atlas, which surrounds the spinal cord (the continuation of the brain) and meninges. The stabilization pattern necessary to hold the head steady is created by the positions of the skull bones and the muscle tension patterns, which determine where the atlas is found. Many people find relief from their headaches through treatments that move the atlas into a central position beneath the skull. They become regular patrons of doctors who move the atlas or therapists who relax the muscles. These treatments are often temporary because the body may need the atlas not to be centered to uphold the skull in the most stable way. *The body will always choose to maintain the most stable structure even if it creates pains in the head. The priority is not to be pain-free but to be stable.* So the painful position of the atlas may be the *best* position for the atlas, in terms of overall bodily function.

Most people with head pressure have not found any relief from conventional treatment. The head pressure is from meningeal tension, and the manipulation of the atlas is usually not effective in relieving meningeal tension. Osteopathic cranial therapy or craniosacral treatment can sometimes give temporary relief.

Every person I have seen with headache, head pressure and migraine has a tilted occiput. (But there are people with a tilted occiput who do not complain of pain.) The tilted occiput causes instability in head balance that is best stabilized by moving the atlas out of a centralized position. The tilted occiput is the cause of the head pain. In theory, effective pain relief should be found by correcting the painful stabilization pattern of the skull/spine. And it is with NCR.

NCR is a wonderful therapy for head pain. It is the best treatment for headaches, head pressure and migraines that I have found.

Heart conditions?

People with heart conditions are safely treated with NCR. However, this is not addressing the cause(s) of the heart condition.

Insomnia?

Insomnia is a condition that is difficult to treat. The causes of it are many, and a good family practitioner has many conditions to rule out. Hormonal problems, allergies, heavy metal poisoning, mineral imbalances, stress and poor home environment are some of the causes of insomnia.

A leading cause of insomnia can be stress, which is often considered to be a *psychological* condition but is very mechanical as well, regardless of its causation. Once present, stress can be relieved very effectively with NCR. Often times the stress can be relieved long-term by the NCR. (*See anxiety*)

Treatment of insomnia is generally biochemical. Sometimes changing nervous system balance with the mineral magnesium or pantothenic acid (vitamin B-5) can be effective. The use of tranquilizers and sleeping pills is usually of symptomatic help, and botanicals such as valerian, skullcap and hops are just a little better. Melatonin, a pineal hormone, tryptophan (now a prescription item) and 5-HTP (a tryptophan precursor) can be symptomatically corrective too.

The use of serine phosphatide salts or the more expensive phosphatidyl serine can be effective because of their damping of adrenal cortisol production. Occasionally, the use of cortisol analogs, like licorice root concentrates, improves cortisol levels, alleviating the need for continued adrenal stimulation to manufacture cortisol and thus allowing the nervous system to rest.

NCR can help to balance the body's hormonal patterns by optimizing nervous system function. Thus adrenal problems like high cortisol levels (a cause of insomnia) can be corrected. Similarly, low estrogen levels, which can lead to insomnia and hot flashes, can sometimes be treated with NCR.

Low energy (fibromyalgia, chronic fatigue)?

Chronic fatigue syndrome (CFS) and the related condition fibromyalgia as well as the general term "low energy" are multi-factorial problems, and part of the condition seems to be structural in nature.

There are many biochemical parameters associated with fibromyalgia and CFS, and they are an important component in a patient's recovery. In CFS and fibromyalgia, treatment of allergies, chronic and acute infections (viruses, bacteria, fungi and parasites), detoxification of heavy metals and chemicals and the correction of problems in the home environment are all important. Treatment of poor sleep, sleep apnea and insomnia is an important consideration as well.

But these are not enough. It is important to realize that there is an additional element to health besides diet and lifestyle, detoxification and treatment of infection, and that is the body's structure. Without proper structure, the brain and nervous system cannot function optimally.

This is why NCR is an integral component for recovery from low energy conditions. With fibromyalgia, the major complaint is the aching of the muscles. The muscles' primary job is to *assist* the skeleton in supporting the body. When there is chronic aching of the muscles, the obvious assumption is that the muscles are overworked because the skeleton is not positioned to support the weight. This is an obvious situation in which to use NCR.

Lymphatic circulation and its malfunctioning, such as lymphoma, lymphatic toxins and lymphoid?

The lymphatic system is part of the body's fluid circulating networks, returning the larger protein and waste products from the cells and tissues. It empties into the circulation at the vena cava near the heart. (The smaller, more watery waste products from the tissues and cells are in the venous blood already.) Lymphatic fluids circulate through the lymphatic system by the contraction and relaxation of the skeletal muscles, moving by muscle actions like frosting squeezed through a pastry tube.

With less skeletal muscle action, there is less movement of the lymphatic fluids. Proper lymphatic function is especially crucial during periods of detoxification like illness, dieting or cleansing programs. When the lymphatic system is not working right, the body can get toxic rapidly. It is sluggish lymphatic functioning that makes the muscles sore, the bowel movements especially foul, the breath smelly, the skin greasy and the temperament sensitive during these times because toxins are backing up in the lymphatic system.

(This is a time when massage can be helpful. There are also home therapy techniques to move lymphatic fluid that you can see in the chapter on immune system function: hydrotherapy techniques in The Naturopathic Dispensary catalog, or read it online http://www.naturopathicdispensary.com.)

The role of NCR for lymphatic circulation is small. There will be a difference in lymphatic functioning, but it will be indirect. The skeletal muscular tone will be different as a result of the postural pattern changes from NCR. This makes chronically tight muscles shorter and more flexible, which promotes lymphatic fluid movement where there would normally be little. There are also changes in nervous system functioning with NCR that could make a difference in the nervous system's response to the toxic situation.

TMD or TMJ (Mouth, head and jaw pains)?

Temporomandibular Disorder (TMD), sometimes referred to as myofacial pain dysfunction or temporomandibular joint (TMJ) syndrome, is a condition involving pain in the muscles of the jaw used for chewing and/or the temporomandibular joint, which connects the lower jaw to the skull. There are limitations in the use of the jaw and joint sounds (clicking, popping or grating noises) when the jaw is used. However, many people normally have such joint sounds in the absence of pain. Pain can spread to the muscles of the shoulders and neck. More rarely, TMD can cause disturbances of vision and balance.

These symptoms are created from the overall position of the bones of the head. Why would TMD occur? The main reason is the position of the temporomandibular joints. When the temporal bones are not positioned symmetrically, the mandible has difficulty making smooth contact with the skull. The temporomandibular joints are then stressed separately and uniquely. When the jaw joint binds, there are joint sounds and often, but not always, pain. The cranial balancing pattern, obviously asymmetrical with the TMD, requires a painful position of the neck bones and musculature to maintain stability. This results in headaches, neck and shoulder pain, jaw pain and even problems with vision. The lop-sided, uneven positions of the temporal bones can lead to balance problems.

I have seen repeated, great results using NCR to treat TMD. The correction for TMD must address the problems of the entire skull, not just the local symptoms. When NCR treatment has progressed and the pain decreases from improved function of the entire head, the patterns of chewing are different. Usually it will be better, but sometimes it can seem worse, especially with bridges, crowns and fillings that are shaped for the mouth of a crooked head.

When poor occlusion occurs, it is important to see a dentist for fine-tuning of the shape of the biting surfaces of the teeth. Continued chewing with a poor bite can traumatize the skull and move the bones of the skeleton into a different, undesirable pattern of stabilization. Rarely dental orthopedics or even orthodontia will be required.

Generally, other treatments are secondary. The use of acupuncture, massage, stress management and nutrition are powerful only as adjuncts to NCR, the fundamental treatment approach for TMD.

(See vertigo and balance problems. See headache, head pressure, and migraine. See sinusitis.)

Multiple sclerosis and amyotrophic lateral sclerosis (Lou Gehrig's disease)? Muscular dystrophy?

These severe conditions affect the nervous system strongly. With MS and ALS, the nerves short-circuit because of unknown changes that affect the glial cells, the fats that insulate the nerves. There is some evidence to suspect infection by viruses, although sometimes they appear to be autoimmune conditions (like allergies). Using NCR to change the brain function and postural pattern fails to address this problem, although it can help the overall function of the body.

My suggested treatment protocol is to emphasize detoxification and nutrition to optimize function of the glial cells. It is especially important is to maintain a very low fat diet. Avoid animal and saturated fats for years (less than ten grams of saturated fat daily), while ingesting at least three tablespoons (forty to fifty grams) daily of vegetable oils high in linoleic acid like olive, sunflower, safflower, soy and flax oils. Eat fish at least three times weekly, being sure to maintain adequate protein consumption on the other days. Consider being animal product free. Take selenium and vitamin E supplements. It can take two years of this therapy to notice improvement, although the worsening of symptoms should slow down sooner.

Muscular dystrophy is a genetic disorder characterized by gradual wasting of the muscles for unknown reasons. I have treated only one person with this disease, and I saw no change in their condition.

Muscle spasms? Neck and shoulder pain?

Muscle spasms and neck and shoulder pain are obvious conditions to treat with NCR. Muscles assist the skeleton to support the body, helping to oppose the actions of gravity. Muscles are tight and painful when the skeleton fails to support the body adequately. Generally, when the neck and shoulder muscles are painful, they are working perfectly. It is the skeletal structure that is so out of position that the muscles have to be painfully tight to help the skeleton hold up the body. In many ways, the muscles and bones working relationship resembles the use of cables to hold up crooked trees in an orchard. The tree would fall over without the support of the cable. No one blames the cable for being tight. Similarly, the muscles need to be tight to support the body because of the skeleton's lack of support. Blaming the muscles for pain from tightness makes no sense.

To correct the muscle spasms or the pain in the neck and shoulder, the structural problems of the body must be corrected. Without correction, the problems of pain and spasms will reoccur. Traditional physical medicine treatment modalities have been shown to be ineffective. NCR is the only treatment technique that has the ability to address the cause of the problem, the poor structural relationship of the body to gravity.

Organ functioning?

The brain and nervous system control the activation of function of the organs of the body. The nutritional status of the body, the toxic load maintained, the general lifestyle, living environment, the history of trauma and the organ damage history all influence organ function. Any person having organ problems needs to pay attention to all these factors while on the road to recovery. NCR can be one factor because the structure of the skeleton affects the nervous system functions, and they control the operating stimulation of the organs.

Orthodontic stress and bruxism (grinding)?

There are a few factors to consider when finding the causes of orthodontic stress and bruxism: personal and nutritional stresses as well as structural problems are worthy of consideration. It is important for a person with dental stress and bruxism to maintain a stable emotional life. It is also sensible to take vitamins, mineral and adaptogenic supplements to minimize the nutritional deficiencies that can put the nervous system on edge.

However, NCR is a very important part of effective treatment of dental stress and bruxism. NCR can relieve the mechanical stress on the nervous system from the musculoskeletal structures, which decreases orthodontic stress and bruxism greatly. Also, some of the effects of bruxism can be reversed. Chronic chewing and grinding affect the shape of the teeth, and as the bite mechanics change, the chewing muscles slowly change the shape of the head. This head shape is rarely a desirable pattern, so NCR can help to remedy the problems created by bruxism and dental stress by reshaping the head.

Incidentally, it is very important for people undergoing orthodontia to have NCR sequences regularly during orthodontic treatment as well as after treatment, because the head alignment patterns created by the orthodontia can be improved greatly with the NCR.

Osteoporosis?

Osteoporosis is a multifaceted disease characterized by excessive bone loss. There are nutritional, lifestyle, hormonal and mechanical factors that affect its progress. Most osteoporosis treatment emphasizes nutrition and medication: supplementation of minerals (especially calcium, magnesium, phosphorus, manganese and boron), vitamin D and hormones (remedying deficiencies of estrogens, natural progesterone or calcitonin and excess cortisol). It is also recommended to stop smoking cigarettes. Finally, weight-bearing exercise is advised.

Cells in the bone known as osteoclasts reabsorb bone, and cells called osteoblasts secrete bone. They are present all the time in living bone, existing in a state of dynamic equilibrium. When the osteoclasts are more active, the area experiences bone loss, and when the osteoblasts migrate into an area, there is bone growth. The assumed mechanism with osteoporosis is this imbalance, with excessive activity of the osteoclasts or a lack of activity of osteoblasts. Hormones are used to correct this imbalance. Certain vitamins and minerals provide all of the nutrients needed to make bone, covering any deficiencies that may exist. Weight-bearing exercise is used because gravitational forces stimulate osteoblasts, while lack of gravity increases osteoclast activity.

NCR dovetails into this picture dramatically because it improves postural patterns. As the postural pattern improves, the amount of weight carried by the skeleton increases. With increased gravitational weight in the bone, the activity levels of the osteoblasts increase. So NCR addresses the gravitational problems of osteoporosis elegantly. Improved posture makes physical activity easier, leading to a further increase in skeletal weight bearing, producing even greater amounts of stronger bone.

Para- and quadriplegics?

Para- and quadriplegics have usually experienced some sort of injury to the spinal cord. At this time, there is no process that regenerates the spinal cord. NCR won't help either, although the other conditions that a para- or quadriplegic has could still be helped with NCR.

Parkinson's disease and tremors?

Parkinson's disease is a condition involving low levels of the neurotransmitter dopamine to specific receptors in the brain stem. The general symptoms of Parkinson's include:

1) Drooling,
2) A mask-like, unemotional appearance of the face,
3) A flexed (tightly hunched) body posture with muscle tightness throughout the body,
4) A limitation of movement generally, including a difficult, shuffling gait when walking,
5) Difficulty standing or with beginning movement (resembling a frozen sort of paralysis) and
6) Visual perception that makes entering doorways and enclosed spaces difficult.

The medical treatment model is to increase the levels of dopamine throughout the brain. Although this is not a cure, it can usually control the severity of tremors. However, the movement and perceptual difficulties do not seemed to be helped with medication. Additionally, the problem for some of the patients I have seen is the side effects of the medication. There is speculation that nutritional supplementation with phosphatidyl serine (300 mg daily) is helpful, but I don't know yet about the efficacy of this. Experimental brain surgeries have been attempted, but the transplanting of brain tissues into the patient's brain has had spotty success.

My clinical experience with Parkinson's disease is encouraging. Generally, I expect to see improvement in all of the symptoms described above. Most of the time, the tremors temporarily worsened with treatment, but in more recent months, with improvements in NCR technique, I have seen less of that.

The reason why NCR is effective for what is considered to be a degeneration of the basal ganglia of the brainstem is that there is impaired circulation of blood and cerebrospinal fluid into this area of the brain for Parkinson's sufferers, and NCR increases circulation. Medications do increase the level of serotonin in the brain, and this resolves the symptom of low serotonin delivery levels in this part of the brain. However, by changing the shape of the skull with NCR, the flow patterns of blood and cerebrospinal fluid are dramatically improved, and this changes the amount of serotonin delivered into the affected areas of the brain too. NCR improves the postural pattern as well, with concomitant greater ease of movement. The perceptual changes observed with NCR seem to revolve around lessening of the mechanical tension in the meningeal system. When this occurs, there is a nervous system-wide improvement in function.

I think that NCR is the most promising treatment currently available for Parkinson's disease. I hope that research money can be found to demonstrate this conclusively.

Phobias?

Phobias are a kind of anxiety discussed earlier in this chapter. They are thinking patterns and behaviors based on exaggerated, irrational fear of a thing or situation. Phobic people are aware that their behavior makes no sense, but it is so unpleasant to experience the fear that they attempt to avoid the situation. Current treatment of phobias consists in behavioral conditioning techniques such as systematic desensitization and exposure therapy. These are often effective but are expensive and time-consuming.

My clinical experience with phobic patients is that NCR treatments make them better. My treatment model explains why phobias are not simply psychiatric problems but are instead ideas created by abnormal brain function, triggered by aberrant flow of cerebrospinal fluid, resulting from the shape of the skull, creating undesirable delivery of neurotransmitters. NCR gradually optimizes head shape as well as the flow and delivery characteristics of neurotransmitters and cerebrospinal fluid.

NCR, then, is a way to cure the phobias instead of attempting to change behavior through counseling and conditioning.

Polio?

Polio is not in the public consciousness much anymore because the use of vaccines has lessened the frequency of outbreaks. For most people infected with polio, the symptoms are like a mild form of flu. But for less than one per cent of the infected population, the sensitive individual can have nerve damage, paralysis and death.

After infection causes nerve damage, the results are permanent. These people experience problems with walking gait and coordination. It wouldn't seem that anything could help, yet I have received reports from my student-doctors that they have had success treating polio sufferers.

The husband of one polio victim described the nightly pain and twitching his wife experienced. After her first treatment sequence, the twitching and night pains stopped. I have never treated a polio victim.

Poor concentration and focus?

Many people complain of poor concentration and an inability to focus their thoughts. It is generally regarded as a problem of inattention or poor thinking habits, at least I always thought so. I was surprised when I found that my ability to concentrate began improving soon after I began treating myself with the endonasal balloons in 1980.

The explanation is the same one used for learning disabilities, anxiety, depression, phobias and other conditions of the brain: After cranial traumas such as birth, falls, beatings, accidents, sports injuries or medical and dental treatment, the bones of the head are not found in their ideal locations. This affects the flow of blood and cerebrospinal fluid in the brain. Compromised circulation leads to varied levels of neurotransmitters in the brain, with some areas getting adequate or excessive neurotransmitter deliveries, and other areas receiving inadequate amounts.

This leads to sub optimal functioning of the brain. In the situation of poor concentration and focus, the brain is not able to perform these tasks because neurotransmitter levels are inadequate. NCR therapy optimizes skull shape, maximizing fluid flow dynamics in the skull, and creating neurotransmitter equilibrium in the brain.

Relationship difficulties?

Manipulation can improve your relationships!? This sounded silly when individuals and couples began telling me so, but I soon came to realize that it is true. Some individuals seem not to get along with anybody, finding something in all of their relationships to blame for their unhappiness. Also couples sometimes are not nice to one another, and they have little tolerance for each another. This breeds poor communication in all of their relationships as well. Such people are often tired, have headaches, sinus problems and snoring, so they just don't feel good.

After undergoing NCR treatment, people feel better. Their brains function better too. They are more tolerant and communicate better with their family and co-workers. One man stopped arguing at work after receiving NCR, although he had previously not heeded numerous reprimands for his constant, ongoing squabbles with his co-workers. One family begged their father/husband to return for more treatments because he was so much more pleasant around the house after NCR.

A woman who had a headache for more than twenty years found herself sexually desiring her husband for the first time in years after NCR rid her of the headache. NCR's improvement in the position of the pelvis can help the quality of couples' sex lives as well. Many children stop behaving aggressively or peevishly after NCR enhances their brain fluids' flow. For some of the children I treat, their behavior with their family and schoolmates determines the frequency with which they are brought in for treatment.

NCR is an important way of improving behavior and relationships.

Sciatica, kyphosis (hunchback), lordosis (swayback), scoliosis (a spiral spine), military spine (from whiplash) and other back problems?

Back problems are the result of the postural pattern of the body leading to excessive stress for the muscles and the nerves, creating pain. Kyphosis, lordosis and scoliosis are postural patterns of the Spine. There is no conventional medical treatment for postural problems until they are so severe that surgery can be used.

Consider a whiplash injury. It is caused by a whip-like action of the head and neck, moving the center of the head forward (anteriorly) on the neck. This makes the head balance differently. The body's solution to the dilemma of holding the head up in a stable pattern is to change the curve of the neck into a straighter or even a reverse curve pattern. No wonder that local treatment of the neck does not help much!

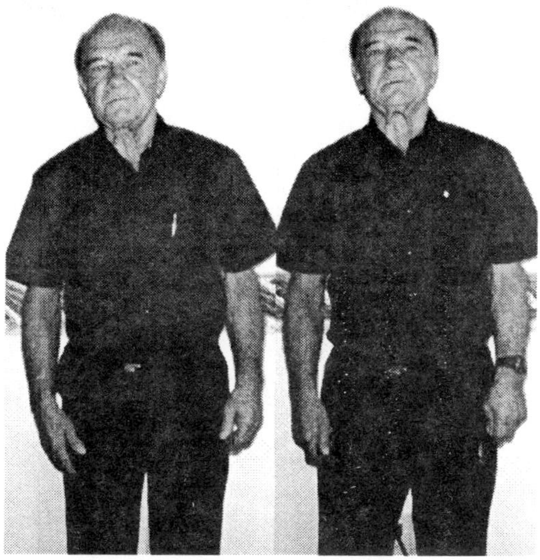

Before After

Similarly, a kyphotic (hunchback condition), scoliotic (spiral-shaped spine) or lordotic (swayback) spine is created from the stabilization pattern of the head. Local treatment of these spinal patterns is without merit. This is why there is generally no treatment for postural problems beyond telling someone to stand up straight. When the bones of the head are misaligned, the only postural patterns that the nervous system can find to support the head in a stable pattern result in kyphosis, lordosis, scoliosis or the whiplash pattern (a very straight spine). Only NCR can routinely expect to make changes in kyphosis, lordosis and scoliosis. This is because the reasons for these postures are not conditions in the spine but instead problems in the position of bones in the skull. It sounds funny to say that scoliosis begins in the face, but it's true!

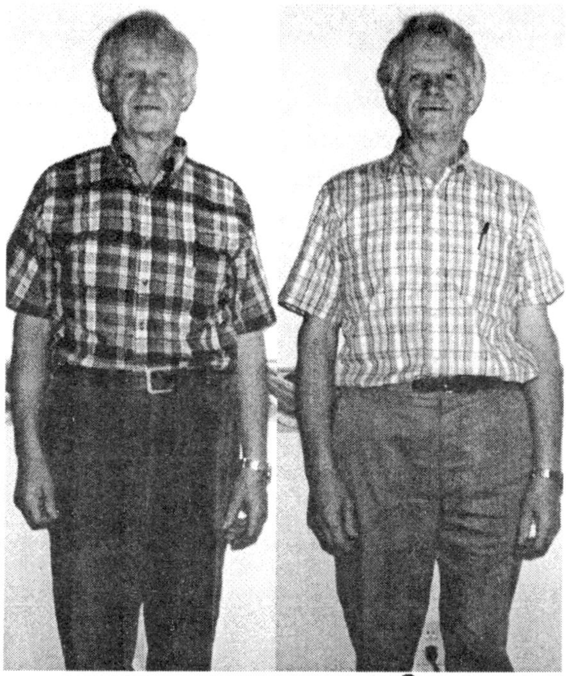

Before **After**

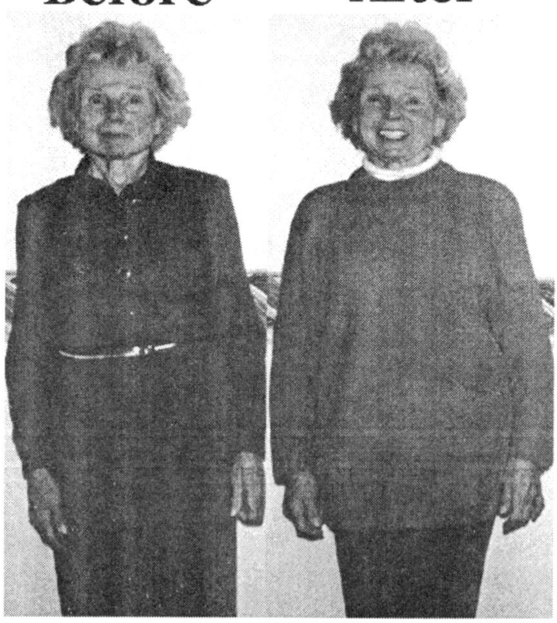

Seizures?

Seizures are rarely cured but are instead controlled. Medications are frequently used, with Phenobarbital, carbamazepine, Tegretol and Dilantin being most prominent. There are nutritional techniques as well: treatment of heavy metal toxicity, hypoglycemia and allergies, following the ketogenic diet and the administration of nutritional supplements such as vitamins B-6, D, E, folic acid, taurine, manganese, choline, betaine, dimethylglycine, sarcosine and selenium all having scientific validation.

Yet the problem of seizures is caused by abnormal activity in the brain where activities are controlled by neurotransmitters. Could it be that changes in neurotransmitter levels in the affected areas of the brain would change seizure activity?

When I first began treating persons with seizures, I had my doubts. With the old Bilateral Nasal Specific (BNS) technique, I would never know what to expect. Sometimes the patients would have seizures on the table, and at other times their seizure frequency and intensity would improve. But any change in the seizure pattern was an indication that I had the concepts relating to the causes of the seizure condition partially correct.

As BNS gradually transformed into NCR, my patients experienced only improvement. This means that neurotransmitter levels are abnormal in persons suffering from seizures, and NCR should become a part of treatment for all such people.

Sinusitis? Sleep apnea? Snoring? Breathing and sinus disorders?

The technique that I first learned using endonasal balloons is called bilateral nasal specific (BNS). The primary intention of the doctors using BNS is to improve breathing and sinus function. (It was only Dr. Stober, my mentor, who realized that there were other treatment objectives for the endonasal balloons.)

When NCR is performed, the endonasal balloon is inflated in one of the two nasal breathing passages one to four times each treatment. The nasal breathing passages (the two areas that begin with the nostrils and end in the throat) are made bigger with NCR (and BNS too). This improves nasal breathing function. As the interlocking bones of the head shift, movement continues throughout the skull until the pressures between the bones are equalized. With BNS, sometimes nasal breathing improvements would last and at other times treatment would be repeated indefinitely. With NCR, most widening of the nasal airways initially created by the endonasal balloon can be retained. NCR enables a person to breathe easily though the nose.

When a person snores, the noisy inhalation and exhalation of air through the mouth creates the noise. It is the chronically clogged or narrow nose and its inability to breathe well that force the need to breathe through the mouth. When NCR opens the nasal airway, the need for mouth breathing is diminished. This diminishes snoring too.

Many people with sleep apnea have terrible problems with the nasal airway. For them, NCR dramatically improves the severity of their sleep apnea. There is less improvement with NCR for the person with sleep apnea, whose tongue falls into the throat, blocking the passage of air down the throat.

Only some of the bones of the cranium have sinuses. The sinuses are caves inside the bones of the head. In some ways, the sinuses of the head are like bathtubs. Bathtubs fill with water and drain through a hole in the lowest part of the tub. When there is a problem with the drain, or if the bathtub is tilted the wrong way, the water stays in the tub. If your bathtub is full of water, it grows scum. One way to keep the slime from growing in the water is to dump bleach into the tub. But the solution to the bathtub problem is to fix the problem of drainage. The symptomatic approach is to control the scum in the water with bleach.

Similarly, each sinus has a small opening, which is usually the lowest area of the floor of the cave. From that opening a small drainage tube leads into the nasal breathing passage. With sinusitis, the drainage area of the sinus is not found in the lowest position. The bones of the head have been pushed into a slight tilt. This prevents complete drainage of the mucus normally manufactured by the mucous membranes of the sinus. If an infective microorganism gets into the area, the mucus is a wonderful breeding area for infection. But the body can kill disease only where the blood stream can touch. The center of a sinus chamber is not part of the bloodstream. Only the walls, floor and ceiling of the sinus are in direct contact with the bloodstream and all its antibodies. When the sinus doesn't drain, the body is capable of only controlling the growth of the microorganism, not killing it off. This is why many sinus infections are chronic: the body can't kill them. The common solution is to use antibacterial substances. Some people use synthetic antibiotics; others use colloidal silver or herbs. Either way, the symptom—the bacteria—is being treated, not the cause—the position of the sinus.

We were not designed to have sinus problems! Our original blueprints did not include sinusitis as an option. As the body optimizes with NCR, the position of the bones housing the sinuses improves, so the sinuses drain better, and the body is able to kill off the original culture of the infection. With NCR, sinus problems stop.

Strokes? Thrombosis (excessive blood clotting)? Left hemisphere paresis?

With conditions like stroke (cerebrovascular accidents), excessive blood clotting (thrombosis) or left hemisphere paresis, my initial impulse is to treat the cause of the condition. Strokes create brain damage and are caused by bursting blood vessels or excessive blood clots blocking the arteries in the brain. So, some strokes are caused by thrombosis. Thrombosis is improved through regular exercise and oral administration of fish oils and gingko.

Controlling blood pressure and maintaining strong blood vessel walls through the use of gingko prevent the other kind of stroke. For this, flavonoids like green tea and bilberry are my choice besides maintaining a low animal fat, adequate protein diet with low levels of simple carbohydrates. (Left hemisphere paresis is a stroke-like condition of unknown origin, so I don't know how to treat this nutritionally.) Manipulation should make no difference in the blood's clotting activity, and I have seen no benefit from NCR. But some of the effects of the stroke and left hemisphere paresis could be mechanical, rather than permanent damage to the brain. In this situation, NCR should be helpful, and it is. Persons who have suffered strokes generally improve their brain functions with NCR. I have never seen a patient with left hemisphere paresis.

Tinnitus?

Tinnitus is a harrowing condition to experience when it is severe. Conventional medical treatment is in its infancy, with competitive noise hearing aids, experimental surgery widening the canal through the bones surrounding the auditory nerve and the administration of sleeping pills and tranquilizers. Changing the relative position of the auditory nerve to its surrounding bones sometimes successfully treats tinnitus.

There are three ways this can be accomplished:

1) The nutritional approach is to use allergy avoidance, reduced inflammation diet techniques, nutritional supplements and detoxification protocols to reduce swelling of the auditory nerve, reducing the interference with nerve function and the tinnitus.

2) Tinnitus suffering can be alleviated with treatment of TMD. How can this be related? It is related because the cause of TMD and some tinnitus is the same—a great difference in the positions of the temporal bones. This leads to pressure against the auditory nerve, causing tinnitus, or can cause poor position of the mandible that leads to friction in the temporomandibular joints (TMD). However, the dental treatment of this situation is indirect because the dentist has access to the teeth and they are mounted in the maxilla, and the contact between the maxilla and temporal bones is the sphenoid bone. NCR treats sphenoid bone position problems more effectively than any other technique.

3) The bones of the skull impinging the auditory nerve can create tinnitus. This is where experimental surgery can be used. Once again, however, this is a wonderful situation for NCR, with less risk and expense than surgery.

I have success with half of the tinnitus cases I treat. Sometimes the ringing in the ears will fluctuate each day. This is not a condition whose ultimate therapy combination has yet been found.

Tuberculosis?

Tuberculosis is an infection with *Mycobacterium*. This disease is on the increase worldwide after many years of relative inactivity. What is worse is that the newer forms of TB are antibiotic resistant. There are studies showing that some botanicals have utility treating TB. Manipulations with NCR will probably make no difference to a tuberculosis infection, but I have never seen a case of TB, so I don't know.

Vertigo and other balance problems?

The only medical treatments used for vertigo and balance problems are medications like Antivert or botanicals like catnip. They are effective only while under the influence of the drug. And they treat only the symptom, not the cause.

Balance problems and vertigo are situations affecting a part of the inner ears known as the semicircular canals. They are located in the bones just behind the visible portion of the ear. The two semicircular canals are each comprised of three bony rings filled with fluid, set at different positions so that at least one of the canals has fluid movement any time the head is moved. The brain uses the six fluid-filled canals to determine where the ground is or at least where the pull of gravity is coming from. The more your head moves, the more the fluid in the inner ear moves, and the more movement the brain is aware of.

The process of determining balance is complex. Each movement of the head causes movement of at least one of the semicircular canals, and the sensors inside the affected canal(s) respond to the fluid movement and stimulate the brain to change body muscle-coordination patterns to react to the movement of the brain.

My clinical observation and experience treating people with poor balance, dizziness and vertigo is that they generally have common structural patterns: The position of their ears is not uniform and symmetrical. When this happens, the brain is using two groups of sensors placed at different angles and heights to determine the position of the ground. Often these people are dependent on their vision to maintain their balance because of this asymmetry.

Consider the complications the brain would encounter if the ears differed in position five degrees and a centimeter (0.4 inches) in vertical (height) position. This would mean that the signal from the inner ears would have a five-degree/ one-centimeter difference in the findings of where the ground is. This would not affect much until the person was walking on irregular terrain, walking on a beam high off the ground, moving in the dark or standing on one leg. In these situations, five degrees of position or one centimeter of height can be very important. I have examined people whose ear positions differ more than three centimeters (1.2 inches). No wonder that they are clumsy!

Imagine what it would be like to be blindfolded and walking with two persons, one at each ear. They are whispering walking conditions to you. What do you do if they give you different information? Do you pick one to believe? Do you stop and get scared? This is the situation a person has when the ears are not positioned symmetrically. Having your ears at different angles and different positions on the head (implying rotation of the temporal bones relative to one another) is a similar experience, except that it seems normal to the sufferer; nobody knows that this situation can be changed!

The normal result expected with NCR is for the temporal bone positions to become more symmetrical. As the ears become more symmetrical, balance (and proprioception) improves.

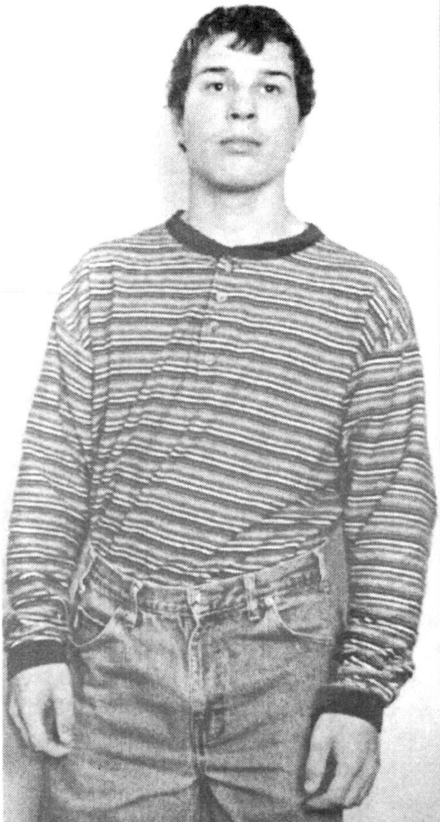

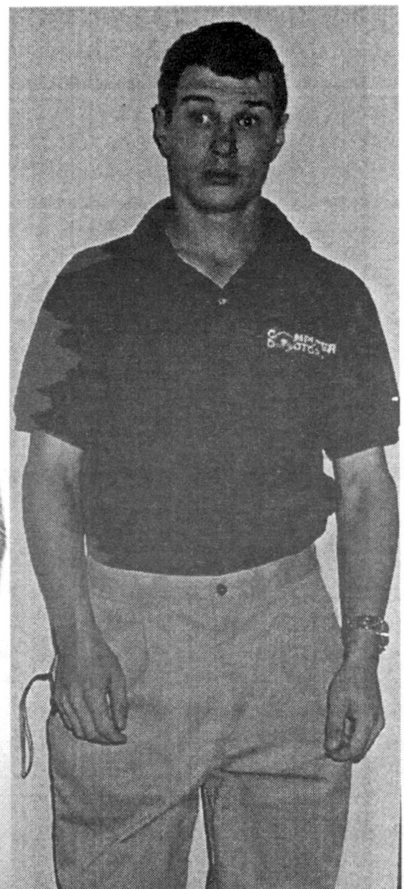

The following text and photos are from a report to an attorney.

Descriptions of Photographs:

The dated photographs you see in the eight-photograph sequence are from my office records. There are six pictures taken before the accident, and the last two are seven and nine months after the accident. The difference in the photos from before and after the accident are notable for the change in format, with the earlier pictures taken with a thirty-five millimeter camera and the later pictures taken with a digital camera.

Mr. Rogers is freely standing in all of these portrait pictures. The changes in the relative position of his head are because of changes in his postural pattern. I took each portrait picture on the day in question. Mr. Rogers' pictures are sized so that his faces in each of the pictures remain approximately the same size. A photo anomaly that made the background appear blue has been removed from the last two portrait pictures. No retouching of the faces have occurred. I apologize for the darkness of the last two photographs (the digital camera has had its problems), but their use was very necessary. They are of great value for this report.

The picture sequence has lines drawn to make observation of the symmetry of each photo and the differences between the photographs easier to see. I drew lines across the bottom of the ears, through each corner of the eyes, and through the corners of the mouth.

Observations:

Please note the gradual changes in the photo sequence. These show the effects of the naturopathic manipulations Mr. Rogers received from me. In the first photograph (taken during his incoming

HERE HE FEELS BAD

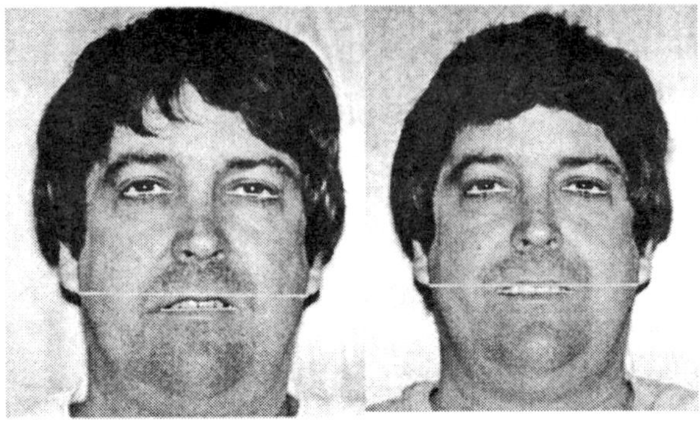

examination), March 4, 1996 March 7, 1996

Mr. Rogers holds his head stiffly erect, tilted slightly forward, with low cheekbones and a crooked nose. By the March 7 photograph, Mr. Rogers already displays a straighter nose, higher cheekbones and a more oval face as well as a more comfortable head position. One of his presenting complaints, sleep apnea, was almost corrected. He had improvement in spinal mobility and a decrease in pain. As the sequence progresses, the gradual changes in facial characteristics and improved head postural position is evident.

WITH EACH TREATMENT SEQUENCE

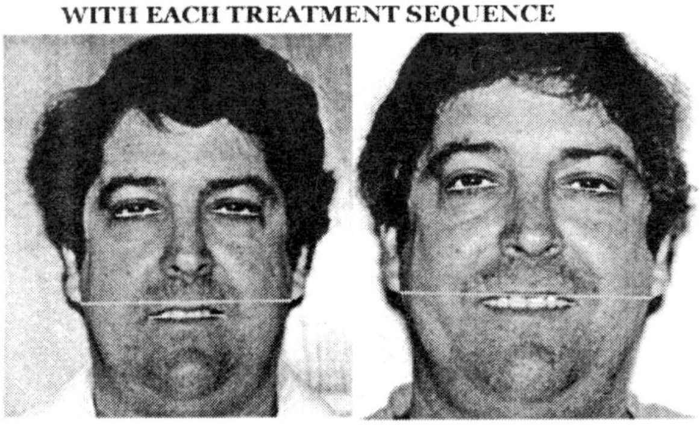

May 2, 1996 August 22, 1996

Similarly, he reported continuing improvements in many facets of his physical actions as well. His chronic neck and back tightness gradually decreased.

HE LOOKS AND FEELS BETTER AND BETTER

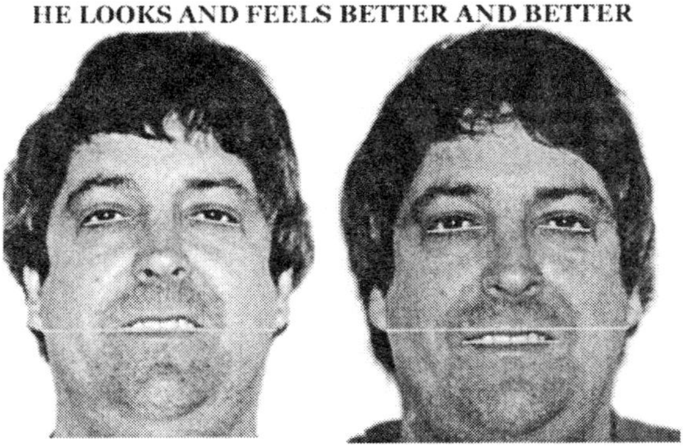

October 31, 1996 December 15, 1996

He was able to stand and extend his arms upward and bend his head backward. He told many people that he had never been able to do this at any time before that.

In the final picture taken before the auto accident, Mr. Rogers looks calm, peaceful and relaxed with a comfortable head position, high cheekbones, markedly different from his appearance on March 4.

Please look again at the same photo sequence, this time noting the lines. The general progression of the photos shows the lines becoming parallel with one another and with the ground as Mr. Rogers' facial symmetry improves.

Soon after the December 15 photograph, Mr. Rogers was in the motor vehicle accident in question. He did not return for treatment until the July treatment sequence. At that time, he had very little improvement of the symptoms that he reported soon after the accident: dizziness, neck and shoulder pain and numbness in his hands and arms.

Even after four treatments (at the time of the photograph), the severe extension of his head is evident, with only some improvement by the September photograph.

Note the slight tilt of the line drawn through the bottom of the ears in the July 14, 1997 photograph. When the ears are found at a tilt like this, the patient will often report dizziness, balance problems or clumsiness.

In the September 19, 1997 photograph, the line is nearly horizontal, and Mr. Rogers reported that his balance was much improved.

AFTER CAR ACCIDENT, HE IS WORSE AGAIN

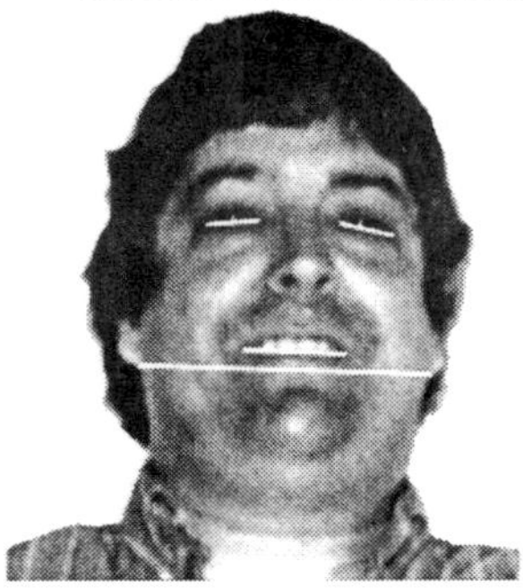

July 14, 1997 September 19, 1997

Here's My Story: Sleep Apnea Cured

By Phillip Rogers

For many years I had suffered from a strange sat of problems EVERY NIGHT for which many doctors had a wide range of opinions but provided no solutions. I would wake up continually throughout the night, often choking and gasping for air to the point that it many times would propel me out of bed and onto the floor. Other times I would experience a short period of total paralysis upon awakening. The doctors had me see "specialists" who were unable to figure out what the problem was. The effects upon awakening also included extreme headaches and dizziness that were so debilitating that it made going to work each morning very difficult. Quite often I would not be able to go to work because it would take many hours until prescription drugs could relieved the problem.

In addition, I was told that I had a deviated septum.

In late 1995 I had a sleep study test where brain and breathing activity are monitored while I slept in a laboratory. The results were very bad. It showed the reason for all my problems. I had a condition called sleep apnea and would stop breathing about

40 times an hour, waking me up continuously. The "specialist" stated that my condition was serious and that I would have to sleep every night for the rest of my life hooked up to a machine that would keep me breathing while asleep. In addition, the "specialist" told me I would probably require surgery that would remove the soft palate area of my mouth.

I was told that people with this bad of a condition were at very serious risk if they did not listen to the experts. Fortunately, I discovered that most people who underwent the surgery still had the problem-minus the removed body parts. I refused that option. God gave us these body parts for a reason!

Also, I was very uncomfortable sleeping hooked up to this machine with a mask covering my face and all the attached tubes. So that was also out of the question. I was facing serious trouble and had no alternative.

Then, through Sam Biser's "The Last Chance Health Letter," I read about the treatments of Dr. Howell. It sure seemed to be a logical approach. He would treat the underlying CAUSE of the problem WITHOUT drugs, surgery, or negative side effects. This was both completely natural and entirely opposite of the "specialists" who only treat symptoms with drugs and surgery, and have a success rate which hovers around zero. (This is shown by the steadily increasing number of Americans whose lives are seriously impaired by this problem every day.)

I first saw Dr. Howell in March 1996. After the first set of his treatments, there was major improvement. During the following 6 weeks I had only a couple of episodes of the apnea and they were very minor. No more total paralysis or gasping for air. About two months after the first treatment I went again and at that point the problem was finally eliminated! Photographs taken before and after even show cosmetic changes. {See the previous article.}

It is now April 1998, more than two years later, and I no longer have any apnea problems. NCR has resolved this terrible problem for good.

NOTE: Since then, I have tried to speak about this with my local sleep apnea group over at the local hospital. Unfortunately, the "sleep specialist", who had a room full of people with breathing machines and masks and/or missing body parts, would not allow me a few words to tell others about this simple and natural technique. It appeared that his only intention was to perpetuate these peoples' suffering and sell machines and surgery and was not interested in any way to relieve their never ending misery. I now believe many of today's doctors need to be tested for a conscience.

Dr. Howell may not be well known, but if you ask ANY of his patients you would begin to realize his technique is something very special. While this treatment has about 5-10 seconds of pain for most people, (for the first few treatments), this may be its strongest testimony. Why would people continue to take time off from work and fly thousands of miles to experience somewhat painful treatments if not for the amazing results? The answer is that they receive improvement that no other technique could ever even come close to. His office is a much different doctor's office, as people are improving and regaining their lives after years of suffering.

Sincerely,

Phil Rogers – Las Vegas, NV

LET'S GET OUR HEADS ON STRAIGHT

Or How My Orthodontic Stress, TMJ and Hearing Problems Got Better

According to Merck's Manual (the bible of the medical profession), sleep apnea syndromes are "a group of potentially lethal disorders in which breathing stops during sleep for long enough periods of time to cause a reduction of oxygen in the blood." There are several possible causes and several treatments suggested, but none as revolutionary and effective as NeuroCranial Restructuring (NCR), which totally handled this serious problem in Phillip, one of my associates and fellow natural healing crusaders.

He suffered from sleep apnea for years, awakening some 40 times each hour. Doctors advised that without a mechanical breathing machine he would probably die. No drugs or nutrition, including his excellent command of herbal healing, was effective.

Then he saw a naturopathic doctor in Tonasket, Washington, who has perfected this unusual therapy, and his sleep became relaxed and restful, and that's not all. His backaches left for good and the treatments even "fixed" his broken nose so completely that a doctor he'd been seeing insisted that he had plastic surgery to straighten it. All he really did was get his head on straight.

The Tonasket, WA naturopath, Dean Howell, tells us, "The skull is like an eight to ten pound bowling ball sitting on top of a pool stick. If the body didn't balance the ball on top, you'd fall over and have to crawl on the ground. Since the body prefers pain to falling over, it will deliberately move the spinal bones (and other organs and tissues) out of place to stabilize itself."

There are actually two problems occurring in the head that force the body to make compensations. In addition to a head that is not centered over the spine, it is also an irregular shape. This pinches and constricts the brain, forcing it to function abnormally slow and somewhat retarded.

"The skull is a container for the brain and the fluids that flow through it." Dr. Howell continues, "There is a small membrane lining the inside of the skull and the brain has to fit inside that. Imagine your brain as a sponge. If you have a round sponge in a square box, there is a squeezing of the sponge and a restriction of the fluid flow within the crimped areas." NCR gives the brain more breathing room to function.

As part of my recent dental surgery, my bite was realigned; correcting a misalignment I had all my life. But, the rest of my body was not ready for correctly aligned teeth. My Eustachian tubes blocked, destroying most of my hearing. It was like trying to hear through gallons of water sloshing around.

Before discovering NCR, I tried everything: herbs, essential oils, massage, chiropractic adjustments, and so on. While some of these treatments were somewhat effective for a while, nothing restored very much of my hearing. I had a 100% blockage in my right ear and 70% in my left.

With Philip's suggestion, I got 4 treatments from one of Dr. Howell's students who were learning NCR in a special Las Vegas class that the doctor was officiating. My left ear opened completely and my right ear improved to 45% or 50% of normal.

These changes were also visible, noticed by my husband — my cheekbones are wider now — and by examination of the ear canal itself.

Then I saw Dr. Howell for my next 4 treatments, about 60 days later. I experienced a return of nearly normal hearing in both ears. I only have an occasional bubbling in my right ear-- the one that was totally blocked after the bite realignment of my teeth.

We believe there is a place for all effective forms of therapy, and you should go to the right place at the right time.

Structural problems must be addressed by structural alignment methods. The arsenal of natural healing gets more complete each day.

Sincerely,

Marge Hartwig

MY SCOLIOSIS IS GOING AWAY!

Ever since I read Sam Biser's words-- "The therapy I have mentioned has no equal in the field of structural healing. It is so powerful that with my own eyes I have seen scoliosis (curvature of the spine) disappear in several months." From that moment I had no doubts that Dr. Howell was going to cure me.

An orthopedic surgeon wanted to do surgery. The possibility of being paralyzed by the surgery was very real. Due to my advanced age of fifty, it was likely that I would not live through the surgery. The recovery period would take many months. I would not be able to work during this time, so there would be financial strain as well.

I had to wait five months for my first appointment with Dr. Howell. My family and friends thought putting balloons up my nose to straighten my back was a crazy idea. I had traveled across the country to see Dr. Howell. I was filled with hope and excitement. When I arrived at the office and saw the stairs leading up to it I almost cried. I have always had to pull myself up stairs. Anyone around thought I was having a heart attack by the time I reached the top. This has been very embarrassing.

Most of my pain occurs at night while lying down. I have not been able to sleep for longer than an hour without waking up in pain. I would have to get up and walk around to relieve the pain. For a long time I have been moody and quick to lose my temper from lack of sleep and too much pain.

I have been to Dr. Howell for five treatment sequences, and with each visit I am in less pain. I can walk up the center of stairs without pulling myself up the railing. I can also sleep for up to four hours now without waking up. When I do wake up I am not in pain. My friends and family tell me I am much more pleasant to be around. I could have gone with surgery and bought my surgeon a new BMW, but instead I went to Dr. Howell and I'm making a down payment on a Chevy. This is the most powerful thing I have done for myself.

Ginny Stafford

WITH NCR, I CAN REALIZE MY FULL POTENTIAL

I am astounded by the way NCR has positively transformed my life physically, mentally and emotionally! After receiving treatment, my spine (crooked since birth and swayback) straightened, feels supple, and my chronic neck and back pain have disappeared. For the first time my weight feels evenly distributed on both legs. There's lightness and a spring in my step.

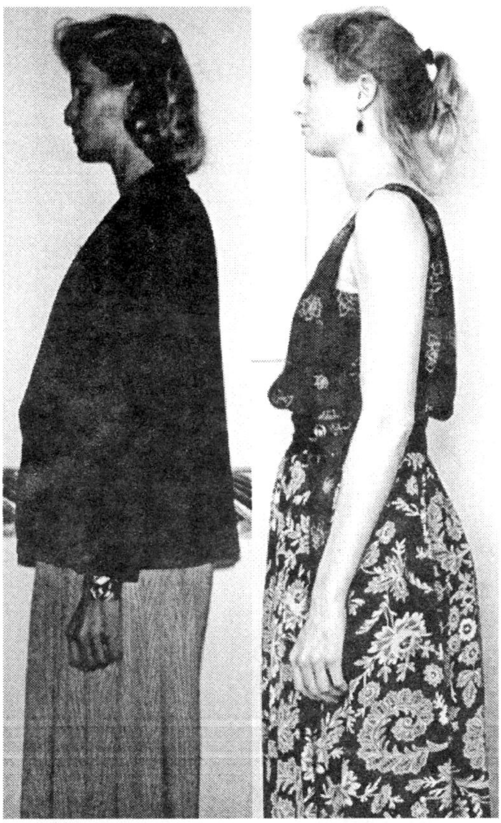

Before After

My chronically stuffy nose has permanently cleared. I need less sleep, have more energy and my face is becoming increasingly symmetrical, well rounded and beautiful.

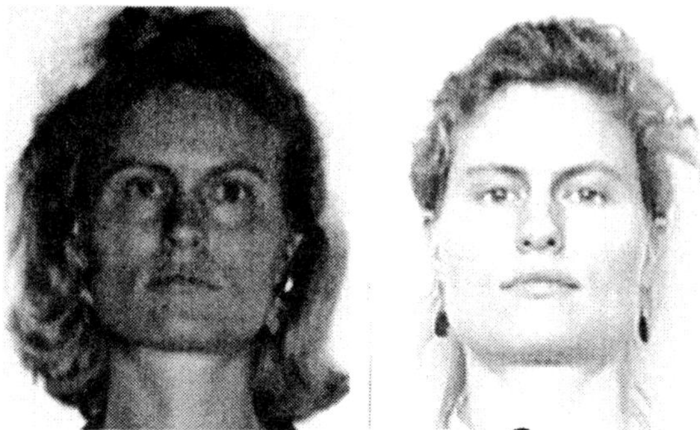

Before **After**

As treatment progresses, I notice that I'm thinking more clearly and calmly. Emotionally I'm also feeling calmer and more secure. My joy and happiness increase with each treatment as my negativity and other baggage from the past melt away. My relationships with others are improving, as I become more easygoing and tolerant. I feel more like my best self all the time, that is, more like the person I most deeply am and was intended to be.

Four months ago I received severe whiplash in an automobile accident, which plunged me into extreme pain. NCR was the only thing that relieved my pain and enabled me to function. Others told me that it would take at least 12 to 18 months for my injury to heal. However, now, after several series of NCR treatments, I feel completely back to normal. My spine and neck are again loose and pain free.

Thank you so much, Dr. Howell! I think that NCR is the greatest gift to humanity in this century. Surely it is the means by which we can realize our full potentials, both individually and collectively. I'm convinced that the world would be amazingly transformed for the better if everyone received NCR.

Trisha Howell

MY TENSIONS CAME FROM MY SCOLIOSIS

Before NCR I didn't realize how stooped my posture was, how unrelaxed I was, and how much I needed to compensate for the structural distortion that resulted from my scoliosis.

One of the early benefits I noticed from my NCR treatments was a profound sense of inner calm that made personal interaction with others naturally more harmonious and that deepened my meditation and martial arts practice. Along with effortlessly improved posture came remarkable changes in my face: eyes less sunken, cheekbones emerging, head held erect, face filling out more the way it was when I was a teenager (forty years ago) and, yes, wrinkles smoothing out.

I look forward to becoming more who I am physically, mentally and spiritually through continued NCR treatments. What a self-discovery!

Sincerely,

Anna Bond, Athens, VT

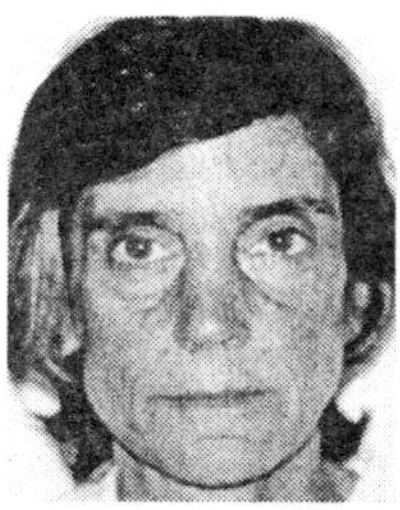

August 12, 1996

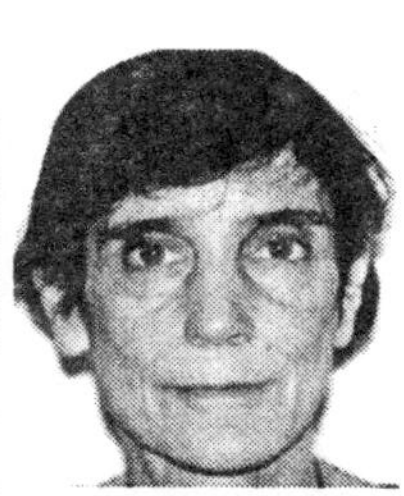

November 21, 1996

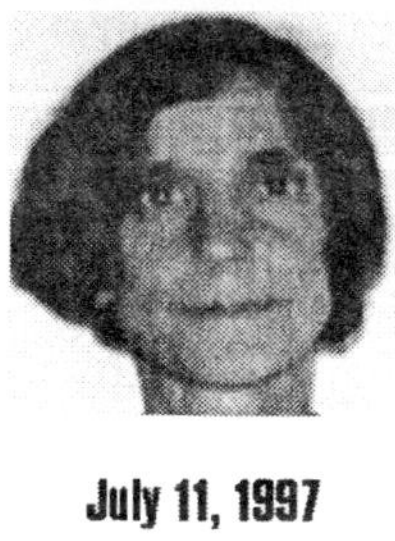

July 11, 1997

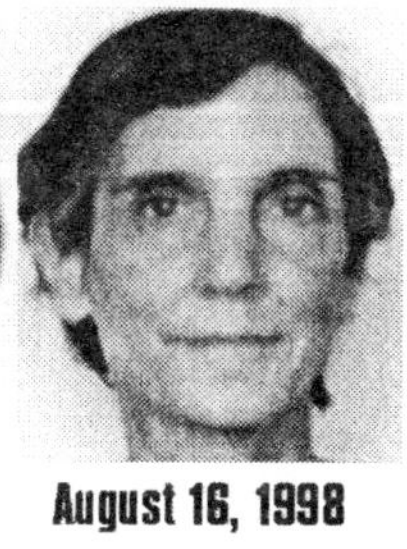

August 16, 1998

MY ANKYLOSING SPONDYLITIS GOT BETTER WITH NCR

Where do I begin?

My condition began at age 17 with a pain in my hip. In one day, I went from the fastest person on my tennis team to the slowest. I deteriorated over the next 5 years. I was diagnosed with Ankylosing Spondylitis (AS).

I went to a neurologist, a rheumatologist, an orthopedist, a chiropractor and a physical therapist for help. All of the doctors and therapists whom I saw clearly wanted to help. However, the diagnosis (with the exception of the chiropractor) was always similar: take non-steroidal anti-inflammatory drugs (NSAIDs) and perform a regimen of stretching contained in a back pamphlet.

The chiropractor was very helpful in increasing my awareness of AS. The MDs correctly diagnosed my condition but did not reveal much information about AS. For instance, it wasn't until six years into the condition that I learned about the process of uncontrolled spinal fusion that characterizes AS.

The chiropractor clearly defined the state of my condition as well as the "what ifs" scenarios for the future. I got manipulations from him three times a week. The manipulations did not help my back but did temporarily increase the mobility in my neck. However, I also felt friction between the vertebrae in my neck. That scared me. I discontinued the treatments.2

I then learned of the Spondylitis Association (SA) and attended a meeting at the National Center for Health. Through SA, my awareness rapidly increased as I met other people with my condition for the first time. I was relieved to meet others with AS and to see that many of them were living happy lives in spite of the physical limitations. But it scared me.

I met a terrific gentleman who was on his fourth hip replacement and was nearly completely fused. When I realized that that was my possible future, I did not like it.

The Spondylitis Association provided a wealth of helpful information. At about the same time, I saw the father of my dearest childhood friend, Charlie Enochs. Jim Enochs took a personal interest in my condition. I consider this one of the most fortunate occurrences in my life. He sent me two nutritional guides, and he recommended various supplements including shark cartilage and fish oil. These are crucial for me. He helped me think about my condition and achieve a better level of acceptance of it. More importantly, he gave me the resolve to keep aggressively fighting the condition.

As my AS management skills improved, I gradually improved my muscular strength close to my former state. However, even with the improvement, I was "locked"' into a slumped position. The pain was perpetual. My neck mobility was virtually gone. With no medical breakthrough on the horizon, I was tempted to accept this lesser physical version of myself.

Although I was not at my lowest physical state, there were additional degenerative signs emerging, including a new pressure pain in the front of my left hip, a constant clicking and popping of my elbows and diminished ankle circulation and mobility. The greatest daily problem was intense tension and corresponding pain in the back of my neck as the muscles strained to hold my head up.

I was experiencing this mental and physical state when Mr. Enochs called and described a treatment that he had undergone in Seattle. He urged me to schedule a visit as soon as could be arranged. He also told me that if it didn't work out for me, he would pay for it, which impressed me greatly.

It took me six months before going to Dr. Howell for NCR. The day before flying to Dr. Howell's clinic, I told Mr. Enochs that a 10% improvement would greatly enhance my life and leave me very satisfied that I attended.

I underwent a sequence with Dr. Howell. A session is a series of half-hour treatments given once a day for four consecutive days. His technique is called NeuroCranial Restructuring (NCR). It really worked for me. Look at my photos!

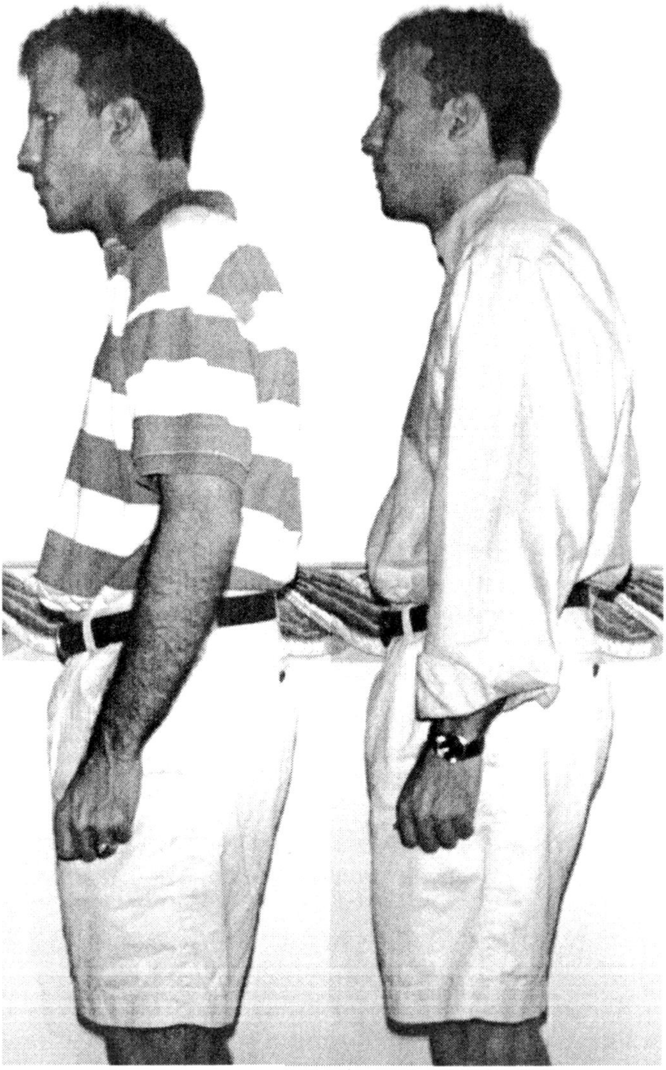

I got:

1) A 60% INCREASE IN ERECT POSTURE!
2) An 85% reduction in pain.
3) A 50% increase in nasal breathing capacity.
4) A 85% reduction in muscular tension in the back of my neck.
5) Between 50% - 75%(at the very least) reduction in spinal scoliosis (i.e.. I now have a fairly straight spine.)
6) A 50% increase in chest expansion while breathing.
7) More than 50% increase in neck mobility.
8) An 85% decrease in the clicking and popping in my elbows.
9) My shoulders are at least 70% closer to their correct position.
10) My pelvis is 70% closer to being on line.
11) My face is a least 30% fuller than it was a year ago!
12) My eyes and ears are more aligned.
13) My nose (which was twice hit over the years) has now returned to 75% of its original shape!

SOME OF THE ANCILLARY BENEFITS OF THIS:

1) I fill out my clothes better because of my improved posture.
2) My pants wear better because of my improved pelvis (i.e. my posterior is fuller).
3) I stand at least an inch taller.
4) My face, not contorted with pain and tension, appears much more relaxed.
5) I walk on the insides of my feet again and my balance is dramatically improved.
6) I am mechanically stronger.
7) My presence in any room I enter is dramatically different.
8) And on and on and on and on and on.

I sincerely hope that this description of my experience will help quantify the potential impact that NCR could have on any degenerative arthritic condition. What is even better is that much of my progress was immediate.

I am only a phone call away from anyone who wishes to ask about my personal experience and results. I can be reached at (404) 843-2224 (phone) or mailto:cuddihy@bellsouth.com (email).

Good luck and best regards for all people looking for guidance and tools to combat any ailment that they are fighting. I am indescribably fortunate to have finally located the guidance and tools for treatment of Ankylosing Spondylitis. It came in the form of Dr. Dean Howell and NeuroCranial Restructuring!

My eternal gratitude,

Jamie Cuddihy III Dunwoody, GA

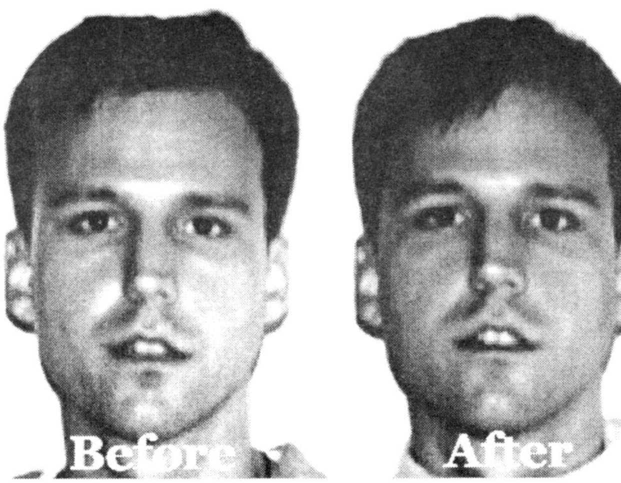

NCR HELPED MY SON'S HYPERACTIVITY AND LEARNING DISABILITIES

Dear Doctor Howell:

Thank you for giving our son back to us! Tucker, our three-year-old, has struggled with interpreting and following through with instructions in the most menial and mundane tasks until his first visit with your gifted techniques of NCR.

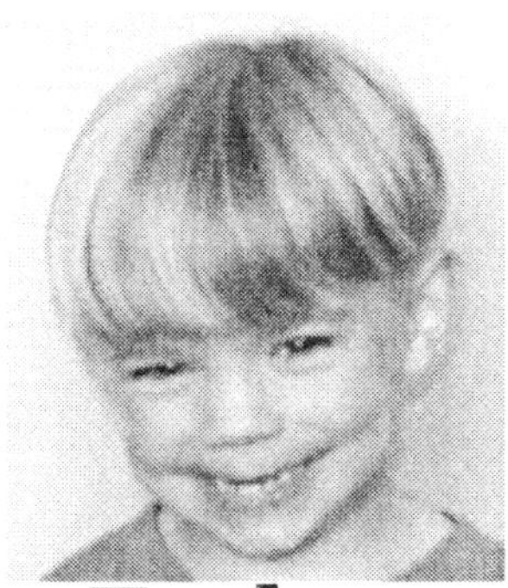

Tucker

After 12 months of trial and repeated frustration, Tucker has finally obtained the opportunity to follow through in toilet training HIMSELF and stay dry, even through the night, without accident or incident.

Where MY son had NO patience for little things like picking up a crayon or marker and drawing or coloring, he now excitedly shows us his pictures exclaiming, "I made this! Isn't it beautiful, Mommy? I made this!"

Every time I think about how his teeth had impeded his ability to speak correctly and caused chewing difficulties, which is now correcting, with the accumulation of repeated NCR treatments, without orthodontics, I give a sigh of relief.

He did NOT have to endure the costly and bothersome surgery for drainage tubes in his ears to relieve a constant barrage of ear infections. The cranial adjustments corrected and relieved his ear pain. It must have been caused by maladjusted bone structure. I CRY tears of joy.

I have to pull myself back from approaching strangers I encounter who have problems in facial structure like I had. I was cured of it, though I was not fully aware the problem until I saw it changing in the sequences of my own before-and-after pictures. I knew that something wasn't even as I would look in the mirror to apply my makeup. I was used to seeing someone that was crooked!

It just feels so much better to go through life being able to stand straight and tall and not have to make a conscious effort to check my posture.

You removed the effects from a head injury that seven specialized medical doctors told me they could do nothing about. It was just something I had to live with. They could find "nothing wrong." NCR allowed me to sleep effortlessly. No more waking to severe inner head pain and throbbing several times a night!

I spent twenty-one years of (sometimes three times a week) chiropractic visits for months on end, spending literally thousands of dollars of my own and so much insurance money, all with the unfulfilled hope of a pain-free lifestyle. I have found that not only does NCR work better, it is also much more cost effective.

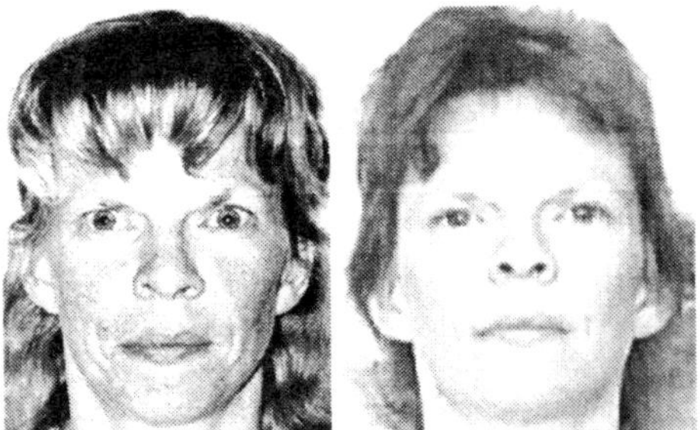

Before **After**

I received complete relief from my pain in only one series of treatments. My posture is corrected; my thoughts are 200-300% clearer, making decision-making a smooth and painless process. There is NO "I should have...." Instead I experience more, "I'm so happy I decided to do that..." which elevates my self-esteem and reassures me that my life is worth living. I am now blessed to be alive, being the one living there; eliminating the severe depression I lived in for years on end prior to receiving your treatments.

In ending, thank you for taking such terrific caring care of my family. Your specialty in medicine puts a new twist on the phrase, "I love balloons" in our household.

Sincerely with gratitude,

Susan Casey (mother of Tucker)
Marysville, WA

MY DOWN'S SYNDROME DAUGHTER GETS BETTER AND BETTER

Dear Dr. Howell,

As all parents of Down's Syndrome (DS) children know, at birth our babies do not look dramatically different from "well" newborns. But as the months and years go by, they develop very slowly and begin to resemble each other more than their parents. Speech, gross and fine motor skills tend to be especially slow to develop.

My DS daughter April, now eight years old, was clearly headed down that road, despite my doing many therapies, programs and natural healing modalities with her. High functioning relative to other DS children, she still had the facial characteristics, droopy posture and slurred speech typical of our kids.

For the past year and a half, however, things have shifted on every level in April as she is blessed to receive NCR treatments from Dr. Dean Howell every three months. April's posture has straightened to near perfect and as a result she excels in her gymnastics practice and skis downhill solo with control from the top of the mountain!

Oh, there have been and continue to be so many desirable changes, both dramatic and subtly cumulative, I don't know where to begin. April's speech is now extraordinarily clear, her thought processes complex. Her natural sense of whimsy can now shine. At last we get to hear her ideas and feelings as she can truly carry on complete conversations.

Her lower jaw no longer projects excessively forward. She no longer has the flat face characteristic of DS people. As the bridge of her nose has come out and we see cheekbones emerge, her eyes have rounded and relaxed into a more

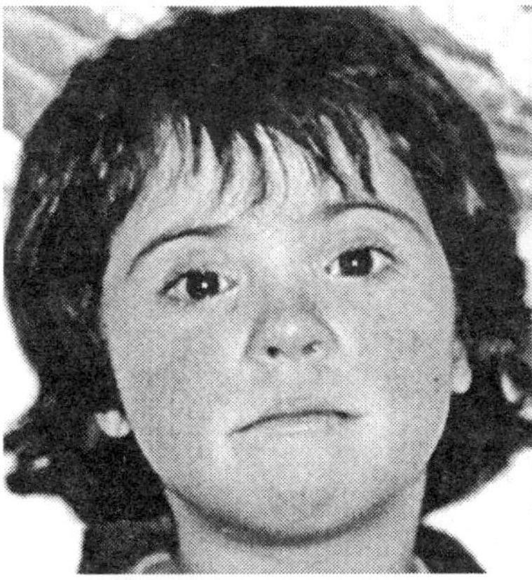

November 18, 1996

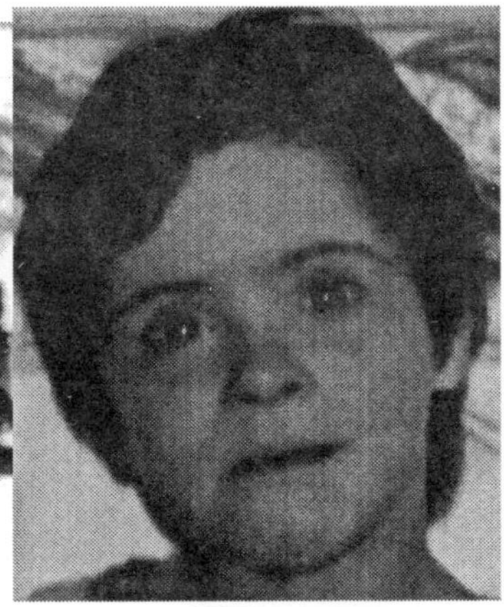

July 14, 1997

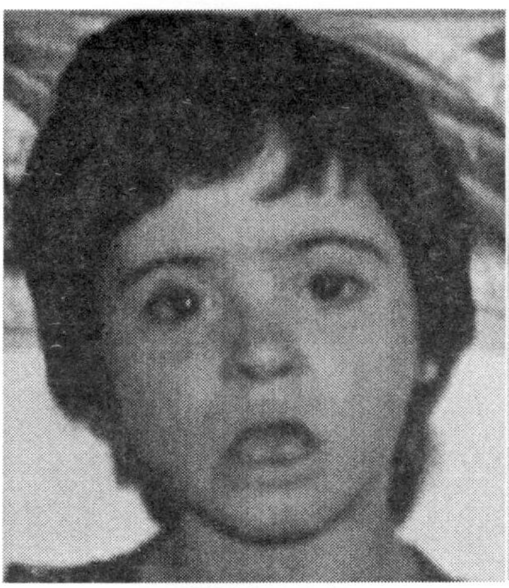

October 20, 1997

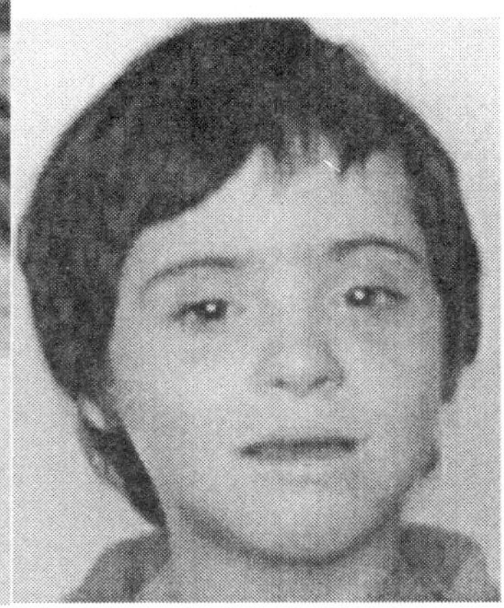

August 16, 1998

natural place. Her lower jaw no longer projects excessively forward. You might not even recognize her as a Down's Syndrome person.

NCR will definitely continue to be part of April's life adventure for years to come.

Thank you, Dr. Dean Howell (and Hillary), for helping to awaken my daughter to her true self.

Anna, mother of April Bond
Athens, VT

MY BIZARRE, BUT PHENOMENAL HEALING EXPERIENCE

by Ginger Chalford, Ph.D.

READ AT YOUR OWN RISK! WHAT YOU ARE ABOUT TO READ MAY TOTALLY CHANGE YOUR LIFE!

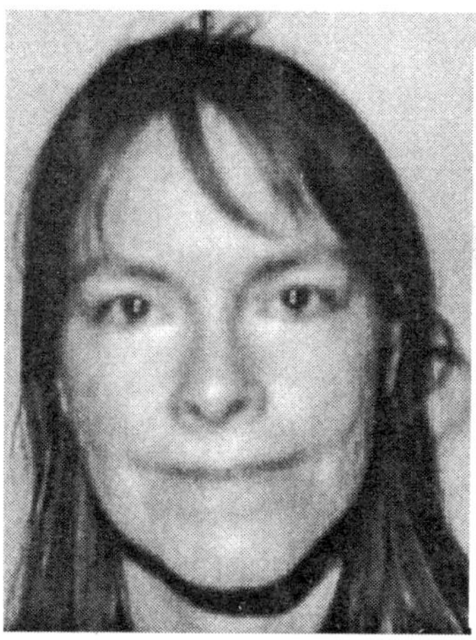
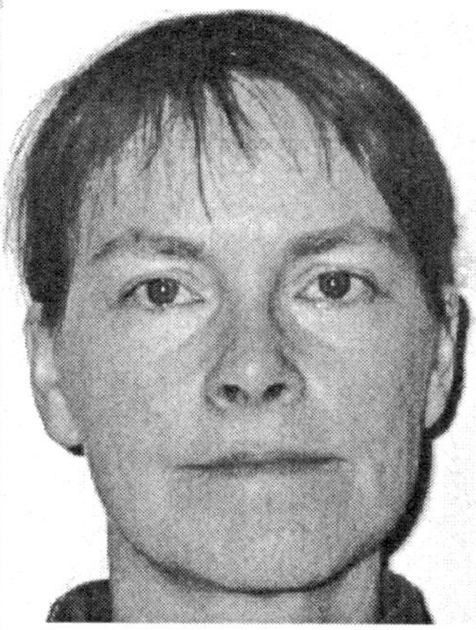
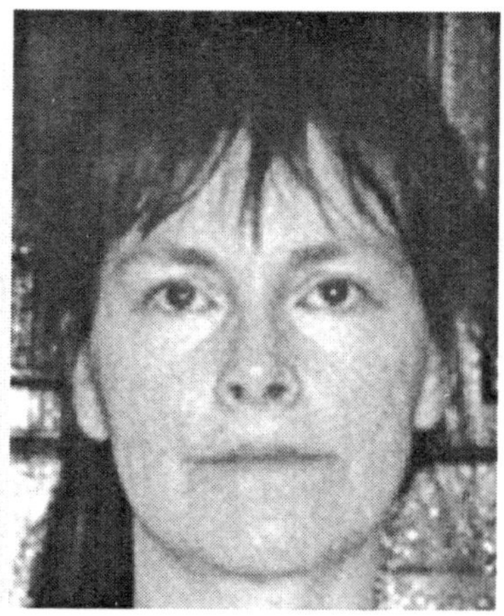

December 10 , 1995 **December 21, 1996** **February 5, 1998**

For several years, I lived with continual pain. Muscles throughout my back, shoulders, neck and head were in continuous spasm. My eyes hurt from unrelenting pressure and my vision was gradually deteriorating.

Sleeping was extremely difficult, because I couldn't find a comfortable position. If I slept on my back, the back of my head would go numb and then hurt like crazy. And the small of my back would aggravate me all day. But if I slept on my side, my shoulder and neck would hurt all day! I would suffer torticolis (wry neck) if by chance a breeze touched the left side of my neck, so I wore scarves and dickeys even through the muggy Florida summer!

Because of the pain and exhaustion due to the pain, I slept a lot. My brain was often on “half function.” I was groggy much of the time. Although I had been a brilliant academic achiever in my youth, I had turned into someone who was confused, absent minded, and ungrounded. I couldn’t work, nor could I create music and art as I’d done years earlier. I was barely functioning.

There were many reasons for this pain, but perhaps the biggest one was that during the 60’s and early 70's, I played violin professionally and didn't hold the instrument properly, hunching up my left shoulder and craning my neck to the left and down. After awhile, this contraction of muscles became permanent, throwing my structure out of balance.

In 1977, I fell backwards onto a terrazzo floor, "cracking" my skull. For months afterward, I had dizziness, and yep, more imbalance. Then in 1986, I had surgery to correct a massive jaw overbite problem and everything got worse, if that was possible. Within a year of the surgery, my little remaining physical comfort became a thing of the past.

My attempts to heal this pain could not include doctors and pain clinics. I simply didn't have the money. I located good Chiropractors, but they gave me only temporary relief. Unfortunately, I was one of those people who could never hold an adjustment. As soon as I'd look up or to the side, "crunch," and I was out of alignment again. My husband, Francois, had to learn how to give me neck adjustments because I needed them several times a day in order to function.

I tried massage therapy too, and it would help temporarily. But then my body would just return to its normal pain and tension within two days, if not sooner. Nutrition helped some, especially the Mineral Toddy, which alleviated my achy joints. Neuromuscular and Rolfing work (with the "finger up the nose" experience) helped a little, and so did some Upledger work. They could shift my cranial plates some, but not expand them outward to relieve the pressure. My muscle pain remained.

Besides researching every alternative health literature source I could find, I knew that there must be a metaphysical reason for all of this suffering. So, I threw myself into years of intensive internal, personal change. My life shifted in glorious, even magical ways, but the pain didn't go away. I prayed for healing every day, and asked for something that could help my compressed cranial bones to relax and expand outward. Laughingly, I would tell everyone that all my problems were "in my head."

Then I received a copy of Sam Biser's "Last Chance Newsletter." In it, he interviewed Dr. Dean Howell, of Everett (before Tonasket), Washington. Dr. Howell shared the amazing results he'd had by doing a therapy currently called NeuroCranial Restructuring, or NCR. This therapy involved moving the cranial plates OUTWARD, expanding the head. He mentioned symptoms that were alleviated by this treatment. TA! DA! They matched mine to a tee! I knew the answer to my prayers had come!

Immediately, I called only to find out that Dr. Howell saw patients only on the West Coast, and so it seemed that, due to the expense, I would have to wait a very long time. But then, Howell's secretary called me to tell me that he was planning a tour, and if I put together enough patients for him, he'd come to Florida. (He no longer does tours, unfortunately.)

YES! Immediately, I became an enthusiastic local representative, telling my friends about this therapy, making flyers about the upcoming visit, and sending interested people copies of the Biser newsletter to read about it for themselves. Anxiously, I awaited the therapy dates. Would it be painful? Would it work? Would it mess me up further? I had my doubts, but they were all put aside because, after all, I'd prayed for this therapy and now it was here. I trusted my gift.

Dr. Dean Howell is a sunny, cherub faced, and charming man. As my husband Francois and I sat down with him the first day of four, he showed us the amazing before and after pictures of people he'd worked on in previous cities of the tour. He told us that the treatment rarely hurt, as there were few nerves inside the sinuses and six nasal passages/chambers (there are 3 chambers to a side). The procedure required that he insert a balloon (actually, the plastic cover doctors use for fingers) placed over a small hand pump into one of the chambers. He would then pump up the balloon, which would open up the locked bones, expanding the head.

A session with him would consist of first determining how one's structure is balance. Then, he would do the insertion and pump where the "opening up" was most needed to unlock the cranial bones. In places of extra lockdown or resistance, he would use up to 10 balloons, as this gave him extra pressure and power. Each insertion/pump would last between 2 to 6 seconds. At the end of each treatment, whether he used the balloon one time or four times, he would balance the whole physical structure. This sounded good, even though I still had trepidation.

Then it was finally time to experience it. How bizarre it was! It felt like plunging into a swimming pool and getting water up my nose. I felt the pressure, and then I felt the bones inside my head give way. It was almost as if a very soft screwdriver bore a hole into the most private recesses of my head.

Nobody had ever been in there before, so at first it felt like a violation of my privacy, my private space. But immediately, I felt an electric surge of energy, as if my whole system was waking up. I breathed a huge, clear breath---amazing! Getting up from the table, I looked at myself in the mirror. My narrow face was wider, rounder. My eyes were set differently and my face was softer - not so angular. Not that tightened look of pain. Again, amazing! I had cheekbones I never knew I had. Obviously, they'd been compressed for so very long.

Then Dr. Howell balanced my spine with a mixture of polarity, chiropractic-like adjustments and energy movement. (The treatments are different now.) I felt energy moving from my head all the way down my spine. He told me that was the freeing of the meninges, which are the fluid compartments surrounding the brain and spinal cord. They naturally determine where the skull and vertebrae sit and balance. When the cranium is locked up, they can't fulfill all of their functions.

The energy and freedom I began to feel with this "energy movement" of my meninges brought me, by the end of my first session, tremendous elation. That was the only way to describe what I felt. I had more bright energy than I knew what to do with, and danced around like a little girl. For years, I hadn't felt this awake and alert so that I had a hard time going to sleep that night. For the first time, it wasn't because of the pain, but because I was so incredibly awake.

The next day we returned for the second session of four. I told Dr. Howell how I felt, and he said not all people have that, only some of them. This day went like the first day, and from this session, I experienced incredible peace and balance. At least my nervous system allowed me to sleep that night, but the pain gradually came back in my head.

I returned disappointed and concerned on the third day. Dr. Howell checked me out and immediate told me that I was still locking up on my right side. So he did extra work on my right side. That night, Francois tested my vertebrae with kinesiology (muscle testing) and for the first time, my atlas and axis, the top two bones of my neck, were “in." The pain was gone and I slept just like a baby - it was wonderful!

The fourth day, we found that the right side was still locking up. Dr. Howell told me that my head had been sitting off to the left - all that violin playing! It was now sitting straighter on my neck. Dr. Howell got my "head on straight" literally! No wonder that no chiropractic adjustment held! In this final session, he discovered that my right side would move and then immediately slide back into the "lock." So he brought out six balloons and went in with more pressure. It really took a lot of strength and persistence, but those bones did give. Like the experience of the first day, this one breakthrough opened me up further. I felt energy rippling through my teeth, all over my head, and my brain/mind suddenly feel light and clear.

Although the basic treatment of four days in a row was finished, the changes in my system had just begun. This is not something to be done frequently. Obviously there are a lot of changes to go through before experiencing a second round of NCR. As of four weeks after the treatment, my head remained centered on my neck.

My Chiropractor commented on how she had no adjustments to make above the third lumbar. Previously, she'd had fifteen or twenty adjustments to make in a session. This time it was only three! She was amazed. She said she wanted to learn the system herself, and I hope she will, for all of South Florida's benefit. After all, there is only one "miracle master" right now, and he's going to get spread really thin around the country as people discover what NCR can do!

Other therapists were excited too. My massage therapist was delighted. A specialist in deep tissue work, she had to really sweat and strain to get into the tissue. Not any more!

My body let her in, down into deeper layers she'd never gotten into before. All the tension gave quickly, which was extraordinary too. Finally, she cleaned all the knots out of my neck and commented, "Your neck is perfect, like a seven-year old. This is the way a neck should be!"

I realized that my body was reflecting my move into a safer reality. After all, my "armoring" disappeared! And the muscles that had been in spasm for almost 20 years no longer held tension. But were they exhausted and weak from all that holding! I could barely do anything for a while without tiring quickly. Now that was a strange feeling, because I had so much physical energy too!

I also returned to get a "fine tuning" from my Upledger practitioner. In the Upledger method, one monitors the rhythm, the pulse or breathing of the meninges. By placing the hands on particular points, like one does in light bodywork, the flow of the meninges, of the structural energy, can be redirected into balance.

She was as amazed as the others. "Your head bones are moving 300% more than before, better than someone who has had the head damage of jaw surgery as you've had!" This session reinforced the sense of inner peace I've had since NCR.

Now I'm sleeping better than in years --no pain! Even around the occipital ridge. The only pain I've been having has come from my structure overhauling itself. Pain comes in for a while in one area, and then the next day moves to another spot.

My husband and I notice that if we hold our bodies in certain off-balanced ways, the pain temporarily returns. This is training us to keep better posture and to pay attention to our bodies' messages! After all, from the metaphysical standpoint, our old imbalanced postures were the physical expression of our negative agendas - our martyr hood, control trips, defensiveness, compromises, and resignations.

The pressure behind and above my eyes has abated, so it is more comfortable to fully open my eyes. Every day has brought some new discovery about my change as my posture shifts to more balance. My muscles, tired or not, show new tone - I feel younger and more energetic and adventurous than ever.

I get a kick out of being mistaken for a 30-something, even though I'm over 50. This may also be due to the "facelift" effect, as my new expanded cheekbones pulled up some saggy skin.

My self-image has improved, and my personality is stronger and more confident. Previously, I'd gone to parties and waited to be introduced, playing shy. In the first party I went to after NCR, I fearlessly held out my hand and introduced myself and met everybody. I didn't realize the difference until afterwards, it had seemed so natural!

My brain function has improved. Before, I had been so scatterbrained that, if I were interrupted, I would forget where I was. Then there would be such a struggle to reorient myself and remember what I had been doing and thinking before, that my life was just hard.

You know, there are lots of interruptions in life! Now, if I'm interrupted, I can simply return to what I was doing and thinking easily, no problem. My concentration and short-term memory is better - I'm remembering people's names and getting more organized!

The changes were not without the accompanying emotional or trauma releases. I'd prepared by having spiritual, emotional, and physical healing work before the NCR. This minimized the resistance to healing as afterwards, I could fearlessly face my issues that new openness brought up.

Others weren't as prepared as I. One woman, who'd had a car accident three years earlier, had to relive the trauma of that event as well as ail the emotional "garbage" that had preceded and triggered it. Another woman I didn't know, but who'd received treatment just ahead of me one day, had to go through emotional trauma relating to her identity as a woman and her relationships with men. Not easy stuff. But you're DONE with it – finally!

For some others, the experience was much easier. My husband Francois experienced a healing of his internal parental drive to please and succeed. He saw slightly better, and had an instant loss of his dyslexia. Now he doesn't have to think about "right" or "left." He just responds instinctively the correct way. He doesn't even transpose numbers anymore. It certainly helps to have the correct numbers if you want to call people back! It saves him the time of listening to his phone messages three and four times just to make sure he gets the numbers right. Life is easier for him now! And, from a wife's perspective, I appreciate his improved good looks and sexy posture.

Our meditations improved as well. We feel it has something to do with the cranial opening, allowing improvement and integration of our brains' functioning. Our temporal lobes, which are involved with emotions and intuitive perception, appear to be in the process of evolving and expanding their functions.

We are both much more intuitive and creative. The new quality and intensity of our visualizations and dreams has especially been rewarding. A sense of electricity, of magic, has seeped into our daily consciousness. Of course, with brain changes, consciousness changes come more easily. This is probably one reason why old emotional traumas release so quickly now.

It has now been four years since my first series of treatments with Dr. Howell. The long-term effect of NCR has been to give me my life back, restore my immune system, and reopen possibilities/Visions/Dreams long closed.

Sometimes, when you look back at your past and its experiences, you'll find one event or marker that stands out as a significant turning point. I have this with NCR, because I can say that my life took a new direction then. I became a new person, gaining new types of life experiences – and finding freedoms lost. If I had not found NCR, where would my pain and languishment have led me?

If it were up to me, I'd require every family to have an NCR doctor along with their family practitioner. Why? Because I know that if I had gotten NCR as a child, I wouldn't have had to have 5 years of braces that didn't work, and musculoskeletal pain that reduces functioning to nearly zero! And I definitely would want every child to get the chance to have the best, happiest, and most fulfilled life.

Now Dr. Howell is not your "regular" doctor. In order to learn more about why some patients have fantastic experiences and others must go through interminable emotional releases to get their healings and realignments, Dr. Howell has done his research. He has traveled around the country visiting other doctors, learning their approaches and looking for insights.

Now how many doctors do you know are willing to do that? Dr. Howell has continued to integrate them into a phenomenally successful system that reduces potential trauma and accelerates astounding healing. After all, if you want the greatest healing effect, go to the cause. And what are more basic that structure, alignment, balance, and brain function? That's why I think Dr. Howell is on to something that is simply stupendous.

It is my feeling that in the future, people won't have to suffer the trauma I have had, due to the exploding numbers of new techniques, concepts, and methodologies becoming available. Integration of these new approaches will give us more elegant ways to heal and change. And Dr. Howell is one of those who are already creating a synergistic path. Believe me, once you have experienced NCR, you'll be able to integrate your life more quickly too! And you'll discover abilities and powers you never knew you had.

Conclusion: This is perhaps the most extraordinary and fast healing method available. Used proactively, it can avoid vast amounts of human suffering and limitation. You'll never know what I'm talking about unless you experience NCR for yourself. And what if you don't? You may be missing a key to your life, your health, and your happiness.

Don't miss this experience.

NCR FOR NEWBORNS?!

by Trisha Howell, MA

The most important and profound medical breakthrough of the 20th century is NeuroCranial Restructuring (NCR). NCR optimizes brain functioning, which is the foundation of our physical, mental, emotional and spiritual well-being.

The brain is like a sponge, saturated with vital fluids. When there is mechanical pressure on the brain from the skull—which is the case for almost all of us—parts of the brain do not receive all the nutrients, hormones, etc. that they need.

NCR unlocks the skull so that the brain can freely expand and function at its full capacity. The skull begins to lock at birth as it is squeezed through the birth canal. Its various bones become compressed and jammed at the sutures and to this extent the meninges—the rubber band-like sack that surrounds and protects the brain—cannot fully expand.

Physical and emotional traumas in any part of the body create a snowball effect, constricting the skull: the meninges tighten and the skull compresses, making the meninges tighten further, etc. When the skull shape degenerates from its original design, the head no longer sits properly on the spine. The spine takes on a distorted shape to support a lopsided head, and the spinal muscles become tight to hold it in place. The muscles function like cables holding up as tree—without this tightness, the person would fall over.

This is why so often massage and chiropractic provide only temporary relief: the spinal distortion and tight muscles are necessary to stabilize an imbalanced head. When symptoms are treated by merely straightening the spine and relaxing the muscles, the body returns to the dysfunctional and sometimes painful position because it's more stable overall.

If instead one treats the cause by restoring the skull to its original design, the muscles relax and the spine returns to its optimal position on its own. Since this is truly a more stable position, it holds permanently (barring more physical or emotional trauma).

NCR is the only therapy that creates permanent, incremental change towards an optimally shaped and positioned skull and spine—and thus an optimally functioning nervous system. This has profound physical effects, such as increased ease, flexibility, energy and mobility as well as relief from a variety of conditions, including breathing disorders, sinus problems, headaches, TMJ, neck and shoulder pain, muscle spasms, scoliosis, seizures, vision problems, whiplash, dyslexia, insomnia, snoring, ear infections, hearing disorders, sleep apnea, Dystonia and Parkinson's tremors.

NCR also has profound mental and emotional effects, such as relief from anxiety, phobias, depression, hyperactivity, nervousness, learning disabilities and even lessening of the effects of Down's syndrome and Alzheimer's. A person feels more relaxed, happy and self-confident. Relationships improve. Learning becomes easier. Creativity is enhanced.

People receiving NCR also report an increased ability to concentrate and focus as well as a greater ease in achieving clarity and insight. Meditators and others who wish to develop themselves spiritually find that NCR makes this much easier and more joyful.

The Age of Aquarius has promised a higher level in human consciousness and well-being. NCR is a significant—perhaps the most significant—therapy facilitating this shift.

Take for example Xander Kriger who began treatment with Dr. Dean Howell, the founder of NCR, at 1 day of age. Xander, who is now 15 months old, has experienced approximately 24 treatments with Dr. Howell. When Xander had his 12-month checkup, doctors were amazed, saying that he was the most neurologically advanced baby they had ever seen. He was put through the tests for 18-month-old children and easily passed. Xander has been walking since 8 1/2 months of age-- child.

Dr. Howell does not believe that Xander is a superbaby but merely normal—unimpeded in his neurological development because his skull is unlocked and exerting no pressure on his brain. Most other children do not develop as quickly, and are functionally impeded even into adulthood, because they don't have this advantage.

Imagine if masses of children and adults received NCR. Our society would be transformed, propelled into an overall higher state of development with the vastly increased physical, emotional, mental and spiritual well-being.

Through NCR we could be happier and more at ease with one another. This would vastly reduce all individual and societal conflict. We would also be sharper mentally and clearer emotionally, making it easier to tackle world problems together and solve them. We would be better equipped with the creativity and insight to formulate a common vision of our future and to implement it.

There is no limit to what we can achieve now—individually and collectively—with optimal brain and nervous system functioning. Our full potential is waiting to be relea1sed with NCR therapy.

RECOMMENDED TITLES

From Howell Canyon Press

P.O. Box 448, Tonasket, WA 98855-0448

(Shipping cost $3.20 per order)

The Original NCR Video (VHS, 1996) $10

Dr. Howell explains his new concepts for physical medicine, with graphics and before-and-after photos.

Unleash Your Structural Power (VHS, 2001) $25

Dr. Howell talks about the newly improved NCR; his staff and patients talk movingly about their experiences with NCR. Includes computerized graphics and a referral list to currently doctors.

NeuroCranial Restructuring: Unleash Your Structural Power—The CD-ROM 2001 $25

This innovative item features all the information found in the third edition of the NCR book and the newer video with computerized menus giving the capability of selecting the text or video information you want from any part of the CD-ROM instantly.

Dynamic Healing Through NCR $13.95

by Susan Stockton

Written by a well-known health writer, this book provides a fresh description of the concepts and applications of NeuroCranial Restructuring.

The Journeying Workbook $12.95

by Trisha Howell

Learn step by step how to internally access an endless wealth of accurate, life changing information that will boost your personal power and positively transform your relationship to everything.

ABOUT THE AUTHOR

Dr. Dean Howell received his doctorate in Naturopathic Medicine from Bastyr University in 1982. His first degree was in mathematics, and he brought a mathematical perspective to medicine that created the quest for simplicity and empirical certainty in healing. Having taken very seriously the Hippocratic oath—which included the injunction to treat the cause rather than the symptoms of disease—Dr. Howell has striven to discover more and more precise methodologies that lead to permanent and cumulative beneficial results. NeuroCranial Restructuring (NCR), which Dr. Howell has been developing for over 18 years, is a powerful and dynamic new approach to physical medicine with broad application. Its effectiveness continues to increase as he incorporates more cutting edge energetic techniques into its operation.

Dr. Howell lives on 200 beautiful wilderness acres in north central Washington State with his wife Trisha and son Derek. When he's not performing NCR and developing it further, Dr. Howell hikes, snowshoes, cooks and plays golf avidly. He is also a voracious reader and a highly creative sounding board for his wife's writing as well as a devoted father.